What Color Is Your
Swimming Pool?

What Color Is Your Swimming Pool?

A Homeowner's Guide to Trouble-Free
Pool, Spa, and Hot Tub Maintenance

Alan E. Sanderfoot

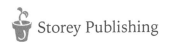 Storey Publishing

The mission of Storey Publishing is to serve our customers by publishing practical information that encourages personal independence in harmony with the environment.

Edited by Nancy W. Ringer
Art direction by Cynthia McFarland
Cover design by Meredith Maker
Cover photographs © D. Boone/CORBIS (front); Downes Swimming Pool
    Company/J. P. Frantz (back)
Text design and production by Susan Bernier
Illustrations by Terry Dovaston and Associates
Indexed by Susan Olason/Indexes & Knowledge Maps

3652 0723 12/07

Storey books are available for special premium and promotional uses and for customized editions. For further information, please call 1-800-793-9396.

Printed in the United States by Von Hoffmann
10 9 8 7 6 5 4 3 2

Library of Congress Cataloging-in-Publication Data

Sanderfoot, Alan E.
     What color is your swimming pool? : a homeowner's guide to trouble-free pool, spa, and hot tub maintenance / Alan Sanderfoot.
        p. cm.
     Includes index.
     ISBN 1-58017-309-8 (alk. paper)
        1. Swimming pools—Maintenance and repair. 2. Spa pools—Maintenance and repair.
     I. Title.
TH4763.S28523 2003
690'.8962—dc21
                                                                    2002154287

Contents

ACKNOWLEDGMENTS

Writing a book of this magnitude is not an endeavor one undertakes alone. Much of the knowledge I have regarding swimming pools and spas I learned during my nine-year stint as editor of *AQUA,* a business magazine for swimming pool and spa professionals. During those years, I met hundreds of intelligent builders, retailers, service technicians, and manufacturers who were kind enough to share their wisdom with me. There aren't enough pages in this book to list everyone who gave me their precious time to make sure I got it right. To everyone who granted me an interview or just took the time to talk shop, I thank you. This book is the result of those impressionable conversations.

A special thanks goes to Nancy Ringer, who edited the manuscript with an eagle's eye and a thirst for knowledge akin to the most inquisitive pool and spa owner.

Preface

When I turned five years old, my top priority was to pass the public pool's swimming proficiency test, which allowed youngsters to advance from the kiddie pool to the "big kid" pool. With its deep diving well, long stretches of water, and sun-bronzed lifeguards, who seemed to make up reasons to blow their whistles at young swimmers — I'm sure it had nothing to do with our countless attempts to get them wet with big, splashy dives — the big pool beckoned to every kid in town. Graduating to the big pool was one of those great summer rites of passage, ranking right up there with shedding your bicycle's training wheels and catching your first fish.

In 1976, when my folks moved our family from that small town to the country, the public swimming pool was no longer easily accessible by bike. So my parents installed a modest pool in our backyard. As time went by, I took on more and more responsibility for maintaining the pool's operation. Before long, I was the one testing the water, adjusting the chemicals, vacuuming the pool, and cleaning the filter. That cool, sparkling water was a constant thrill for me, and so, strangely enough, I never minded these chores very much.

While in college, I paid my tuition bills in part by working as a swim instructor and lifeguard. A good tan was still a hot commodity on college campuses back then, and I welcomed the opportunity to develop mine.

After graduating with a degree in journalism, I was fortunate to find work at several magazines before landing a job as editor of *AQUA,* a trade magazine for swimming pool and hot tub professionals. For nine years I developed articles and seminars to help pool and spa professionals improve their businesses and better serve their customers.

Now I find myself writing a pool and spa care book, and I'm glad to have the opportunity to work not just with pool and spa professionals but also with pool and spa owners. Much of what I've learned over the past decade or so has been poured into this book. I've come to realize that most pool problems are easy to fix if you understand how pools and spas are built, what characterizes a properly plumbed filtration system, and how to achieve perfectly balanced and sanitized water. I've tried to deconstruct these issues in this book, explaining not only how pool and spa equipment works but also how to choose, maintain, and repair it. After reading this book, I hope that you'll feel intimately familiar with the operation of your pool or spa and the maintenance steps necessary to keep it in tip-top shape — the only prerequisite to carefree enjoyment of your aquatic paradise.

Introduction

America's backyards have never looked better. No longer simply a place to host family picnics or watch birds at the feeder, the backyard today is being landscaped and designed with all the amenities of the best resorts. At the top of most homeowners' wish lists are pools and spas, which bring the soothing sights and sounds of water to the yard while providing an idyllic setting for entertaining, socializing, relaxing, and exercise. However, the well-outfitted yard might also include a barbecue grill, an outdoor fireplace, multiple furniture groupings, a sound system, landscape lighting, patio heaters, and children's play equipment. As we embrace the outdoor living lifestyle, we're making our yards as useful and functional as the family room or kitchen.

The theme trumpeted by the design community over the past few years has been "What's in is out and what's out is in." As designers started to bring stone, glass, and metal furnishings into the home, luxurious fabrics and upscale furnishings began making their way outdoors. Today, the boundary between the house and the yard continues to disintegrate as trend-setting designers incorporate the same, or similar, materials indoors and outdoors. This design technique breaks down the barrier between interior and exterior and gives the feeling of a larger home.

The trend toward comfortable backyard living originated with the "nesting" phenomenon of the 1990s — a time when dual-income families were so exhausted at day's end that they couldn't muster the energy to leave their homes in search of relaxation and fun. Family values were making headlines, and parents (often divorced) were grasping for unique ways to bond with their children. Meanwhile, empty nesters were reaping the rewards of a healthy economy and cashing in those CDs to redo their homes with entertainment systems, professional-grade kitchens, and luxurious bathrooms inspired by decadent health spas. This trend is continuing as an increasing number of baby boomers retire and start to spend their life's savings on their homes to make them *the* place for children and grandchildren to visit. Oftentimes, this means adding a pool or spa environment to the outdoor living space.

The idea that you can create an aquatic paradise in your own backyard is appealing for many reasons. Above all, it allows you to maximize your limited leisure time in the comfort of your own home. But a pool and spa also make it

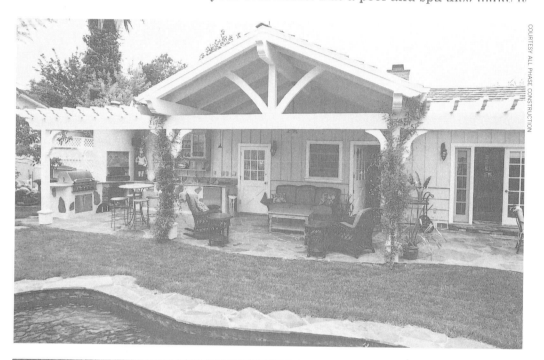

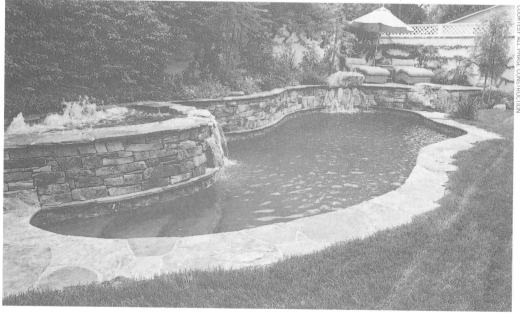

Outdoor kitchens, like the one pictured at top, are growing in popularity as more homeowners seek to create elaborate outdoor rooms to accompany their pools and spas. This project includes a wood-burning oven and multiple seating areas around the pool *(bottom)*.

easy and convenient to engage in aquatic exercise, heralded for being low-impact while offering moderate resistance for strength training. In fact, new aquatic exercise equipment is introduced every day — from aquatic dumbbells and jogging belts to underwater treadmills and rowing devices. Pool and spa owners who want to take their aquatic workout to the next level might opt for a pool with a swim jet, which provides a current of resistance you can swim against, thereby making any pool suitable for "lap" swimming. The same effect can be achieved by purchasing a fitness spa, which is large enough for stationary swimming but offers the added benefit of hydrotherapy.

Speaking of hydrotherapy, it's the number one reason people purchase a spa. Hot-water hydrotherapy is known to lessen stress, relieve muscle soreness, and promote better sleep when done about an hour before bedtime. And with the addition of special spa fragrances now on the market, spa users can enjoy the soothing benefits of aromatherapy along with their hydrotherapy.

According to landscape designers and builders, the cost to "furnish" a yard averages from 10 to 15 percent of a home's value. For example, if you have a $200,000 home, you can expect to pay at least $20,000 to $30,000 for a complete pool and spa environment. If you have a $2 million estate, then $300,000 for a pool and spa area may not be a ridiculous budget to consider. Clearly, the ideal pool and spa for someone in the middle of the economic scale is quite different from that for someone at the upper end. Nevertheless, even those with only a moderate household income can create a backyard that will be the envy of the neighborhood. It just takes imagination. Instead of an indoor pool lined with tile mosaics, your budget might be better suited for an aboveground pool with custom decking. Instead of an outdoor kitchen with a wood-burning pizza oven, you may have to settle for a stainless-steel gas grill. Likewise, you may have to forgo the multiple furniture groupings you saw at the designer showroom and head on down to your local patio furniture retailer and see what's to your liking and on sale.

Whatever you do, don't let cost alone get in the way of creating your ideal pool and spa oasis. With your imagination as your guide, you, too, can transform your backyard into an outdoor room of your dreams, with a pool or spa as the focal point.

With that said, the rest of this book will focus on the pool and spa element of backyard living, with particular attention paid to the operation, maintenance, and repair of pools and spas. Nevertheless, remember that to fully enjoy your pool or spa requires an investment in your total backyard environment. After all, what good is a pool if you don't have a comfortable chair for poolside lounging? What good is a spa if you don't have landscaping lighting to lead the way to your midnight soak beneath the stars?

1 Choosing the Right Pool

Shopping for the perfect backyard swimming pool can be as mind-boggling as shopping for a new car. The choices of make, model, and accessories are just as overwhelming, and advice from competing salespeople often seems contradictory and confusing.

Clearly, much has changed since the 1950s, when simply designed swimming pools began to speckle American backyards like blue diamonds dropped from the clouds. Today, thanks to new technologies and advances in construction, the ubiquitous rectangle and kidney shapes have given way to free-form lagoons and vanishing-edge designs.

Though the wealth of options available has made shopping for a pool more difficult and confusing than ever, at least one thing is clear: If you can dream it, there's some designer out there who can help you build it.

In this chapter, we'll look at the various types of pools available today and discuss the basic pros and cons of each. Understanding the various types of pools will not only help you choose one that's right for your home, region, and budget, but also help you better understand how to maintain it.

THE POOLSIDE LANDSCAPE

If you think honestly about how you plan to use your pool, you'll quickly realize that you'll be spending a lot more time *around* your pool than in it. Whether you're hosting a poolside dinner party or simply lounging in a deck chair on a day off from work, most of your poolside hours will be spent enjoying the atmosphere of the pool environment, rather than swimming. As more and more homeowners and pool designers come to this realization, we see many more pool designs incorporating water features and lighting to capitalize on the sensual, aural, and therapeutic relationship of water in our lives. As you discover the wonderful sights and sounds of water, don't be surprised if you agree to budget as much money for the landscaping *above* the waterline as you do for the pool structure *below* it.

To help guide you on your path to poolside pleasures, all you need is the advice of a trusted professional, either a landscape designer or a professional pool and spa builder. These experts are listed in the phone book, but be sure to ask for references, browse through portfolios, and check out actual job sites before signing on the bottom line.

With any poolscape, the major design considerations are water features, decking, landscaping, and lighting.

Water Features

Water features contribute to a truly spectacular poolscape. Depending on the design, they can bring drama and excitement or tranquillity and serenity to an aquatic environment. Countless options are available. Sheeting waterfalls that cascade like curtains of liquid glass are popular; the noise they create is soothing, and kids love to stand beneath them and get drenched. To tie together a pool and spa, you might consider installing a spillway that runs from a raised spa into the pool below. Consult with your pool designer to explore the full range of options available in your space and on your budget.

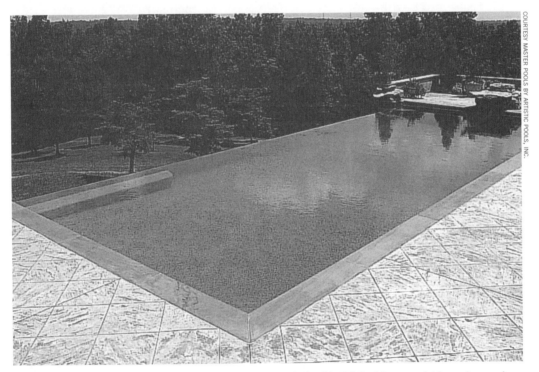

COURTESY MASTER POOLS BY ARTISTIC POOLS, INC.

A blue aggregate pool surface reflects the passing clouds in this 50-foot-long vanishing-edge pool, which is surrounded by a stamped-concrete deck that resembles cut stone pavers.

Decking

The material you choose for your pool deck does for the pool environment exactly what new flooring — whether carpeting, wood, tile, or stone — does for a room in your home: It creates a mood and sets the tone for the type of activity that will take place there.

Poured concrete decks are still commonplace, as are the cement coatings that help keep concrete cool enough for bare feet despite summer's unrelenting sun. But if you really want to create a comfortable and inviting outdoor living space, you may want to invest in something that will be enjoyable both to look at as well as to relax upon. Brick or stone inlays can dress up a gray concrete deck without adding too much to the cost. Of course, all-stone or all-brick decks provide the most luxurious setting. If you want the look without the cost, consider stamped concrete, which can be colored and embossed to resemble your favorite flagstone pavers or antique bricks. Plus, if you can mimic in the pool deck any stonework used in the home construction, your pool area will tie in seamlessly with the rest of the home and more closely resemble an outdoor room.

Landscaping

Like frosting on a cake, landscaping elevates something already wonderful to new heights. But landscaping is much more than mere window dressing. The right trees and shrubs not only create a natural enclosure but also serve as a windbreak that reduces evaporation and heat loss in your pool and makes swimming more comfortable. Perennials and annuals can add a needed splash of color and soften the harsh edges of an otherwise barren poolscape. The options are endless.

When planning your pool's landscape, consider the following:

~ Plant trees where they won't drop many leaves into the pool (unless, of course, you like the idea of spending endless hours with the leaf rake removing fallen leaves from the water).

~ Use shrubs and trees to create a windbreak, but if you plant them along the fence line, make sure that children won't be able to climb the trees as the plantings mature and gain unauthorized access to the pool area.

~ Use large container plantings to bring in masses of colorful flowers and green foliage onto the pool deck. Containers add height and a sculptural element to your poolscape.

~ Talk to your builder about building natural-looking planters into your pool design. Built-in planters can simplify your gardening and ensure that your plantings contribute to the overall pool aesthetic.

- If you're using lots of rocks in your pool design, incorporate strategically placed plants to soften the look and make the rocks appear more indigenous to the landscape.
- Pick plantings wisely to make sure they're suitable for your pool environment. Most plants don't thrive next to hot, sun-drenched concrete or when splashed with copious amounts of chlorinated water.
- If your budget permits, install a drip irrigation system hooked up to an automatic timer to ensure that your landscape investment doesn't die if someone is not around to water it for a few days.

Lighting

If you think of the last time you saw a play, concert, or other stage performance, you know how important the lighting was to the overall set design. Well, the same concept applies to a backyard pool. If you want to enjoy your pool beyond daylight hours, you'll need to incorporate sufficient lighting. However, resist any inclination you might have to simply mount large floodlights on the back of your house and point them toward the pool. Instead, work with your pool designer or landscape planner to create a nighttime setting that would impress even the most demanding Broadway producer.

To achieve dramatic effect and useful illumination:

- Uplight trees.
- Illuminate pathways and changes in elevation, such as steps.
- Spotlight fountains and statuary.
- Use underwater lighting so swimmers can see the pool bottom.
- Point fixtures away from the house so that you're not looking into a bright bulb when you view the pool from the home.
- Use perimeter fiber-optic lighting to frame the pool or highlight special features, such as sheeting waterfalls.
- Choose fixtures, sconces, and shades that complement the overall backyard design.

ABOVEGROUND POOLS

Aboveground pools come in a variety of sizes, though their shapes are limited to circles, ovals, and rectangles. For many years, these pools were relegated to the low end of the pool hierarchy because they were inexpensive and provided few design possibilities. Though they remain the least expensive pools you can buy (some cost under $1,000), they now offer greater durability and more design options than ever before.

An aboveground pool is basically a 48- or 52-inch-high (122 or 288 cm) wall with a vinyl liner. The walls are most often made of steel or heavy-duty polymers, but some are made of wood. The bottom of the pool is usually lined with a bed of sand to provide a smooth surface on which the liner can rest. Either the liner hangs over the wall and is locked in place with the pool's top rail or it has a beaded edge that feeds into a track system around the pool to keep it from slipping down.

Aboveground pools must be installed on level ground. Most are not designed to be installed below grade, so every attempt should be made to keep excavation to a minimum. Site the pool or excavate your yard so that rainwater will run away from the pool and not settle around it.

Many aboveground pools are sold as a kit that includes all of the pool equipment a homeowner needs to get the aboveground pool up and running. If you feel handy and your yard requires little excavation, you should be able to install an aboveground pool, with the help of a few friends, in a weekend. (For

DESIGN TIPS FOR YOUR ABOVEGROUND POOL

Up until the mid-1990s, aboveground pools had a reputation for being little more than oversized tin cans rusting away in the backyards of America. But now that depiction is far from true. New advances in design and construction have made aboveground pools as aesthetically pleasing as many in-ground pools.

To make your aboveground pool the envy of the neighborhood, consider these design tips:

- Treat your backyard like an exterior room of your home, and plan the placement of the pool with as much care as you would the new entertainment center you purchased for the family room.

- Aboveground pool walls come in scores of colors and patterns. Select one that complements the design of your home and garden.

- Coordinate the pool's color scheme with your outdoor furniture, shade umbrellas, house trim, and other backyard features to help it blend in with the surroundings.

- To camouflage the pool walls, plant shrubs and flowers around it.

- If your yard slopes, install the pool into the hillside and surround it with wood decking for an in-ground-pool look.

- Position the pool for maximum sun exposure.

step-by-step instructions, see How to Install an Aboveground Pool, page 173.) You can also have your aboveground pool installed by professionals for a few hundred dollars. Most specialty pool dealers offer this service or can recommend a contractor for you to use.

A unique variety of aboveground pool is the portable pool, which either is inflatable or has an easy-to-assemble PVC framework that supports a thick vinyl shell. Unlike the more traditional aboveground pools, these inflatable and vinyl-walled pools can usually be assembled quickly and enjoyed in the same day.

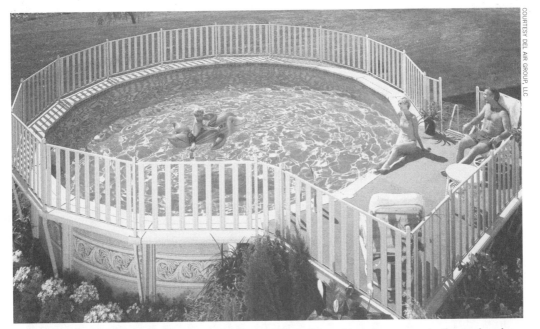

This aluminum pool is beautifully landscaped. A small deck provides easy access to the pool and a perfect spot to lounge and supervise children.

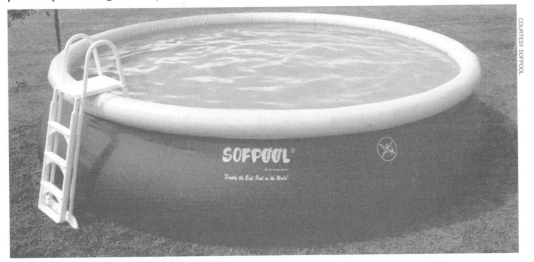

Vinyl, or soft-sided, pools have the advantage of being inexpensive and portable. Pools with PVC frames are also available, ensuring rust-free ownership.

ON-GROUND POOLS

A unique hybrid of aboveground and in-ground pools is the on-ground pool, which is a manufactured pool that can be installed completely aboveground, completely below ground, or partially below ground. It gives homeowners the option of purchasing a pool that's less expensive than a traditional in-ground pool while having a pool with a much lower profile than that of a traditional aboveground pool.

IN-GROUND POOLS

In-ground pools can be as plain as a loaf of white bread or as creatively complex as a seven-grain sourdough baguette. What you choose will depend largely on the size of your pocketbook and how much customization you'll demand of your final design. Because of the excavation, plumbing, and electrical requirements of in-ground pools, they should be installed only by trained and licensed professionals.

An in-ground pool can be vinyl-lined, fiberglass, or concrete.

Vinyl-Lined Pools

When vinyl-lined pools were first introduced, they put pool ownership within financial reach for thousands of families. Their uniform construction made them easy for pool builders to install, and consumers could purchase a pool with the confidence that "what you see is what you get," which isn't always true with a custom concrete pool design. In fact, vinyl-lined pools earned the moniker "cookie-cutter pools" because the early designs were limited by size, shape, and liner colors — meaning one vinyl-lined pool looked very much like the next. They were also called "packaged pools" because they were typically sold as a complete pool system that included the walls, liner, and equipment — everything an installer would need to build the pool.

Today's vinyl-lined pools, however, can be as customized as their concrete counterparts. That's because the steel or polymer modular wall panels can be configured to create an endless variety of shapes, and the liners themselves — which can be 20 to 30 millimeters thick — can be custom fabricated to fit any pool shape and size imaginable.

Here are a few more advances in vinyl-lined pool construction worth noting:

~ **Vinyl liners.** Long gone are the days when solid blue or white liners were the only choices for pool owners. Thanks to advances in printing

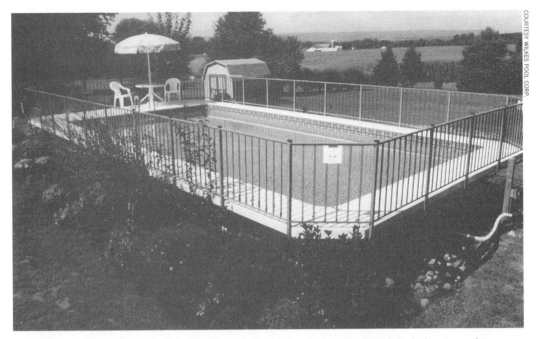

An on-ground pool is essentially an aboveground pool that is installed partially below ground to achieve more of an in-ground-pool look.

technology, vinyl liners can now be made to resemble realistic-looking tile, stone, and myriad other patterns. You can choose from an array of aquatic colors and patterns to achieve just the look you're after, whether that's a woodland pond, Caribbean lagoon, or pebbly beach.

~ **Steps.** In days gone by, you could identify a vinyl-lined pool by its steps, which were always white and tended to stand out like athletic socks worn with a blue suit. For many designers, this fashion faux pas was enough to keep them from working with vinyl-lined pools. Fortunately, there are now ways to disguise the steps and make them blend in with the rest of the pool. One option is colored steps; the color can be coordinated with liner patterns. Another option calls for installing the liner right over the steps, which creates the continuous surface appearance you get with a custom concrete pool.

~ **Coping.** Another telltale sign of a vinyl-lined pool used to be the white coping that surrounded the pool. The coping system secured the liner in place and provided a frame for pouring the concrete deck. Vinyl-lined pools are now often built with cantilevered decks — that is, decks that overhang the pool slightly. This type of deck design can be constructed from concrete, stone, or brick. It hides the coping and creates a more finished look. Coping that accommodates perimeter fiber-optic lighting is also available for vinyl-lined pools.

Vinyl-lined pools are often less expensive than concrete pools, making their cost more easily justified, especially if you live in a climate where the summer swim season is just four to six months long. And with all of the design features now available, you don't have to worry about giving up aesthetics when purchasing a vinyl-lined pool.

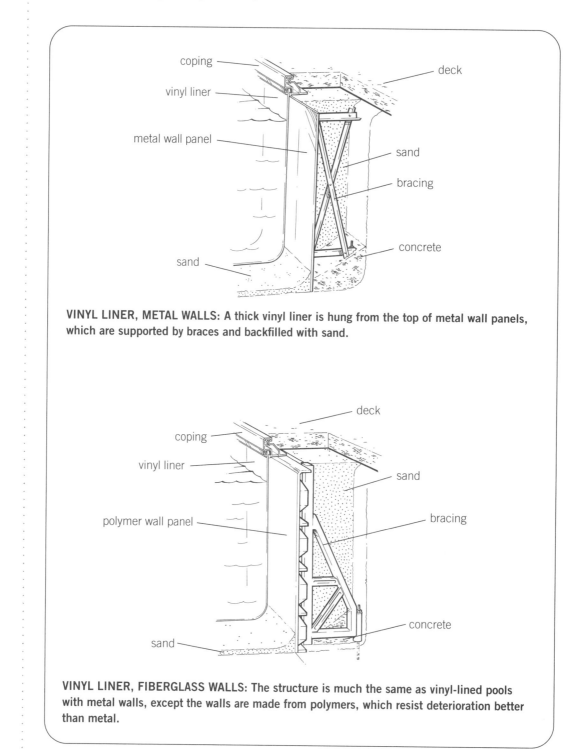

VINYL LINER, METAL WALLS: A thick vinyl liner is hung from the top of metal wall panels, which are supported by braces and backfilled with sand.

VINYL LINER, FIBERGLASS WALLS: The structure is much the same as vinyl-lined pools with metal walls, except the walls are made from polymers, which resist deterioration better than metal.

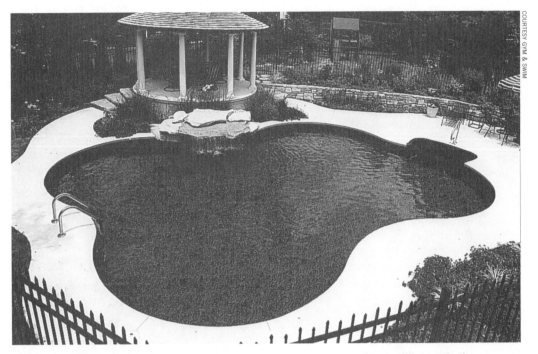

A dark liner, black steps, and a rock waterfall give this vinyl-lined pool a pondlike aesthetic.

Fiberglass Pools

Fiberglass pools are a one-piece reinforced fiberglass shell. When delivered to a job site, the shell is carefully positioned in an excavated hole. Sometimes this involves carefully craning the shell over the house to get it into the backyard. So it's important to consider the cost to deliver such a pool to your job site and whether or not you have adequate access to position the pool in place. If you have a waterfront home, you may be able to arrange to have the pool floated from a more easily accessible location across the water to its final resting spot in your backyard.

The one-piece, molded construction of the shell means that the pool you choose will be exactly the same as the one you get. Plus, the installation of a fiberglass pool is faster than that of a custom concrete pool. And the smooth fiberglass surface is less likely to harbor algae than a plaster pool surface.

Like a vinyl-lined pool, fiberglass pools can have cantilevered decks for a more custom look. Color selection is limited to white, blue, and a few earth tones, but the look can be customized by installing ceramic tile along the waterline. Fiberglass pools are most commonly installed in the ground, but they can also be installed on the ground or on rooftops or decks that have adequate support. In some locales, fiberglass pools have even been *floated* alongside docks in natural waterways, where they provide safe swimming in the otherwise murky waters of lakes, bays, and inlets.

All of this means that a prefabricated fiberglass pool may end up costing you *more* than a custom concrete pool.

Each fiberglass pool manufacturer offers a catalog of pool shapes and sizes, increasing the odds that it has something to suit most pool buyers' needs. But if one manufacturer doesn't have something you like, shop the others, who will have a few different shapes and sizes from which to choose.

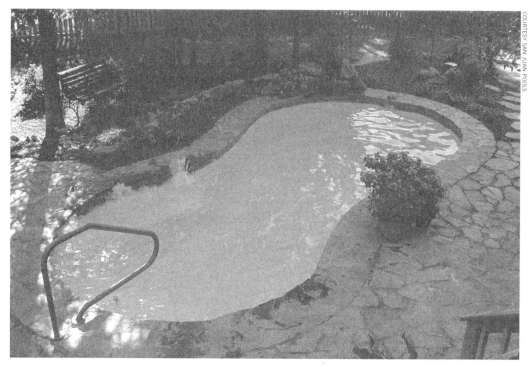

This one-piece fiberglass pool looks custom-designed thanks to cantilevered flagstone decking and captivating water features.

ONE-PIECE FIBERGLASS POOL: A one-piece, molded fiberglass shell is lifted from a truck and lowered into the excavation site, where it is meticulously backfilled with sand to ensure that there are no air pockets that could damage the shell.

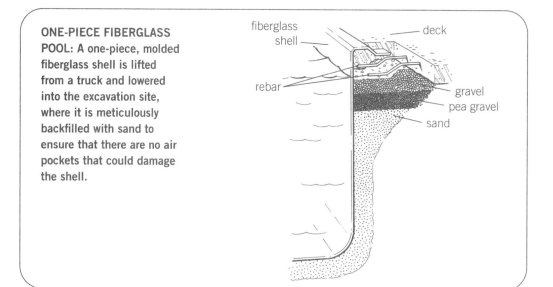

Concrete Pools

For the greatest design flexibility, you may opt for a concrete pool. Manufactured entirely on-site, the design of a concrete pool is limited only by one's imagination and the artistry of the craftsmen working on the project. Concrete makes it possible to achieve everything from artificial rock outcroppings, streambeds, and grottoes to underwater benches with therapy jets, fountains, and other amenities. Though builders and designers can achieve some of these effects with vinyl-lined and one-piece fiberglass pools, the vast majority of designers turn to concrete when they want to create a unique and truly inspirational waterscape for the home.

Regardless of the shape and size of a concrete pool, the process of building it is predictable. First, engineering plans are drawn up. The pool hole is then excavated according to those plans. Next, the hole is lined with a skeleton of crisscrossing rebar. Then concrete is sprayed over the steel latticework. Sprayed concrete can be either gunite (an almost dry mix of sand and cement) or shotcrete (a wetter form of gunite). Spraying the concrete helps ensure that every area of the pool gets equal and sufficient coverage. Concrete can also be poured, but this requires the use of special concrete forms inside the pool hole. Spraying is much easier and, thus, a much more popular method of application.

After the concrete cures, which could take days (depending on the thickness of the concrete and the dampness of the climate), a finishing surface is applied. Why is a finishing surface necessary? Though the concrete vessel is itself waterproof, its surface may be rough, which could promote algae growth. Plus, concrete isn't as attractive and versatile as the finishing surfaces, which include plaster, paint, stone aggregate, fiberglass, and tile.

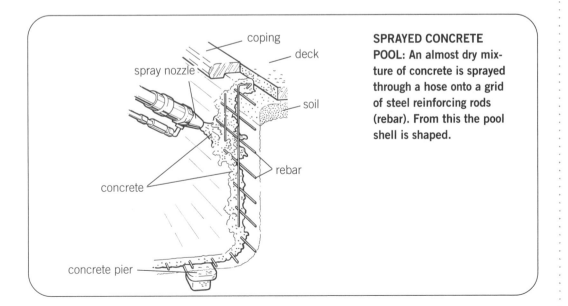

SPRAYED CONCRETE POOL: An almost dry mixture of concrete is sprayed through a hose onto a grid of steel reinforcing rods (rebar). From this the pool shell is shaped.

Stress cracks, also called crazing, will appear in plaster walls that are not cured properly. When you finish a pool with concrete, you must fill the pool with water immediately, because the plaster hardens and cures best under water. Proper water chemistry is also imperative for plaster-surfaced pools. Poor water balance can lead to pitting of the plaster surface, turning a wall that was once as smooth as a beach ball into something that's as rough as a coral reef.

Plaster. This is the mother of all pool surfaces, with a long, much-lauded history of success because of its versatility and functionality. Pool plaster can be white or colored, and it's troweled over the concrete shell to create a waterproof surface that's as beautiful as it is practical. Plaster is usually complemented by an array of tile at the waterline, just below the coping. The tile makes a nice finishing touch and provides an easy-to-clean surface at just the spot where water and scum deposits are most likely to form.

Paint. One of the cheapest pool surfaces, paint also has the shortest life span. However, many pool owners like paint because it allows them to "redecorate" their pool every few years. Many colors of marine-grade paint are available for pool applications, making it possible to cover your pool with geometric designs, murals, or whatever your imagination dreams up. Paint is not a good option in areas with a high water table, however. If you empty your pool — as you must in order to repaint it — in an area with a high water table, the ground water pressure may pop the empty shell right out of the ground. (For more information on painting pools, see chapter 16.)

Stone aggregate. If you're after that "carved-from-nature" look of a pond or lagoon, stone aggregate is the pool surface of choice. These polished pebbles are mixed with an epoxy and troweled over the concrete pool shell, creating a waterproof surface that looks natural and is pleasing to the touch. Manufacturers of stone aggregate have mixed and matched numerous color combinations, making it possible for you to achieve just the look you're after, whether it's the aquatic green of a Caribbean beach or the midnight blue of a mountain lake.

Fiberglass. Often used as a resurfacing agent for renovated pools, fiberglass can also be applied over a new concrete pool shell. The result is a smooth, waterproof surface with the same benefits of one-piece fiberglass pools described earlier.

Tile. If cost is not a factor, you may want to consider tile for your pool surface. Though tile is the most costly pool surface, it's also the easiest to maintain. Plus, you can incorporate incredible design details, including custom mosaics and inlays. Even if you don't desire (or can't afford) a completely tiled pool, you may want to plaster the pool and then include tile inlays on the steps, walls, and floor to add a touch of sophistication or whimsy.

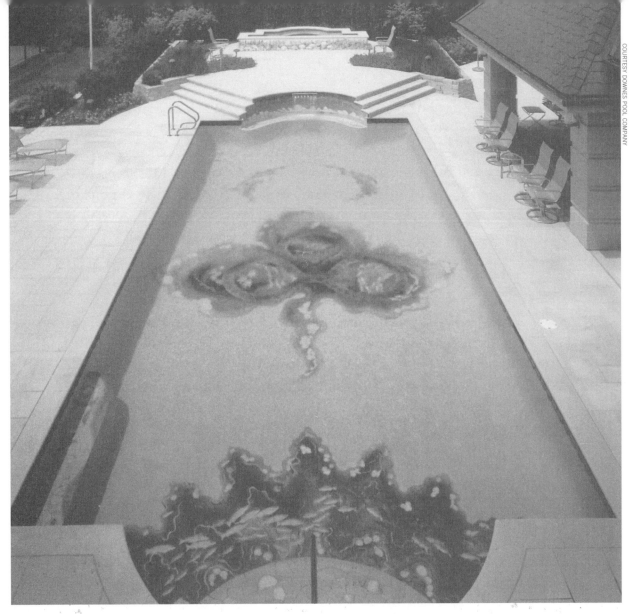

An intricate tile mosaic brings a sense of artistry to this beautiful pool and spa installation.

SELECTING A SITE FOR AN IN-GROUND POOL

Planning a swimming pool installation can be a daunting task. That's understandable, because unlike a piece of furniture, a swimming pool can't be moved to another corner of the room if you don't like where you first put it. Also, there are a host of building codes and regulations that restrict where and how you may construct a pool. Fortunately, your pool designer and builder can help you determine the best location for your swimming pool to maximize your enjoyment and keep expenses down.

When you're ready to get started, make a list of the following considerations. Research each carefully. The information you dig up will aid you through the planning process.

Building Restrictions

Study the zoning and building laws for your property. Zoning laws usually dictate how close to your property lines construction can take place. To ensure that your neighbor's yard isn't flooded with runoff from your new pool deck, there may also be restrictions on how much of your yard can be covered with decking and in which direction it must slope. Also, many municipalities require that pools be fenced in. As with most building or home improvement projects, you may need a building permit before work commences.

Water Restrictions

Some municipalities prohibit the use of city water for filling swimming pools, usually because of drought conditions that have forced their city councils to make rulings regarding acceptable water usage. If you live in such an area, you'll have to make arrangements to have water delivered to your site when the pool is completed. Also, some municipalities prohibit pool owners from discharging their pool water into the city's sewer system. If that's the case where you live, you may want to opt for a pool that has a cartridge filter system so you don't have to *backwash* the filter to clean it. During the typical backwash cycle, pool water is reversed through the filter to dislodge debris and the dirty water is diverted to a waste line leading to the sewer system.

Soil Conditions

Until you test your soil, you won't know what type of construction costs you're likely to incur. Sandy soil, expansive soil, rocks, and other ground factors all present unique building concerns you'll need to discuss with your contractor. A high water table, in particular, can drastically increase construction costs because a drainage system needs to be installed to keep the site dry during construction of the pool shell. Knowing this ahead of time can save you a lot of aggravation and expense down the road. It can be difficult to test the soil yourself, so plan to hire a soil engineer to analyze your soil for you. A soil engineer can also tell you how high your water table is before you start digging.

Utilities

Gas, electrical, telephone, cable, and water lines may need to be relocated to make room for your pool. The cost of relocation will depend on which utilities you're working with and how far the lines need to be moved. There's also the cost to have utilities run to your pool equipment and the surrounding landscape, including plumbing, electrical, and, if you have a gas heater, gas.

Many communities offer free "dig-safe hotlines" that you can call to schedule an appointment to have someone visit your home and mark where the lines are buried. If you don't call and then you hit a utility line during excavation, you most likely will be liable for the cost of repair.

During construction, your pool builder will coordinate with an electrician to take care of any electrical concerns.

Site Access

Heavy machinery will be needed to dig the hole for your pool, and this equipment needs easy access to your job site. Ideally, the pathway should be stable and at least 8 feet (2.5 m) wide. Where access is limited, you can use smaller machinery and wheelbarrows to remove the soil. However, as you might expect, this greatly increases the construction time and the cost of the final project.

Landscaping

Pool construction takes a heavy toll on established landscaping. Before you begin, discuss with your builder the impact construction will have on surrounding trees, shrubs, plants, and lawn so there are no surprises. To reduce the cost of removing excavated soil from the site, consider using it to create berms, elevated decking, raised water features, and other unique landscape details.

Equipment Location

In your excitement to find the ideal spot for your pool, don't forget to consider where the equipment — the pump/motor, filter, heater, chemical feeder, etc. — will go. Ideally, pool equipment should be within 50 feet (15 m) of the pool and no more than 2 feet (0.6 m) above pool grade to ensure proper priming of the pump. With this in mind, you'll want to find a place where the equipment will be out of sight and the sound will be muffled. The equipment should be placed on a level concrete pad, with plenty of room around the equipment for someone to make repairs comfortably.

Pool Access

When positioning your pool, consider how swimmers will access the water and make sure the siting is appropriate in terms of both convenience and safety. A pool placed near a garage could entice some children to jump in from the roof. Most small children want to enter the water at the first edge of the pool they come to, so that area should be the shallowest. Consider the flow from the house and changing room to the pool area to make sure it's direct and clear of obstructions. When designing the deck and landscaping, do whatever you can to discourage people from walking across lawns on their way to the pool, which will track dirt and grass clippings into the water.

Diving Boards and Slides

Diving and sliding require a certain minimum depth of water to ensure safety. Diving is especially problematic. If the diving well is too shallow, a diver can hit his or her head on the bottom, causing spinal cord injuries.

Because each pool has its own unique diving configuration and each diver is physically different, it's difficult to determine what is a safe diving depth for all divers in all pools. Any recommended safe diving depths you may come across in your research will be based more on industry standards than on physical science. I mention this here because a pool with a diving well costs much more than a pool without one, and many builders will try to keep a sale by recommending the shallowest diving well possible. My advice is that if you must have a diving board, don't skimp on the diving well.

Even if you opt for a diving pool, keep in mind that most diving accidents occur in 3 feet (0.9 m) or less of water. In other words, most diving accidents occur where diving was never intended.

Views

There are two main reasons to consider the view of your pool:

~ You want a clear view from the most likely vantage points for the adults who are supervising children.
~ You want to be able to enjoy the gorgeous view of your poolscape from around the yard and from within the home.

The logistics of viewpoints is extremely important with vanishing-edge pools, in which one or more sides of the pool appear to be missing and the water seems to spill into nowhere (for an example, see page 5). The illusion is created by lowering one or more of the pool walls and allowing water to spill into a catch basin on the back side, where it is then circulated back into the pool. If the pool isn't positioned correctly, you might be able to view the catch basin from the second story of the house, thereby spoiling the illusion. Your builder or design professional can help you draft a site plan that will show how your pool can be viewed from different areas of your home.

Solar Matters

Unless you live in the desert or the rain forest, you probably want your pool to receive as much direct sunlight as possible. Maximizing solar exposure will not only reduce your pool heating costs but also provide more hours of sun-drenched swimming. To make the best use of the sun's rays, the pool should have a southern or western exposure. You can harness more of the sun's energy by having a dark-bottom pool (which absorbs heat) as opposed to a light-bottom pool (which reflects heat).

Though you want to maximize the pool's exposure to the sun, you also want to create shady spots where poolside loungers can escape the unrelenting rays. Trees are nice, but the leaves that fall from them can mean you'll be spending more time with a leaf rake in your hand when you'd prefer to be holding an iced tea. As an alternative, consider awnings, umbrellas, gazebos, and arbors.

Windbreaks

One of the greatest causes of pool water evaporation and cooling is wind across the surface of the water. Not only does wind increase the cost of operating a pool, excessive wind can make poolside lounging unpleasant. The simple solution is windbreaks, which can be created naturally with trees and shrubs or architecturally with walls and fences.

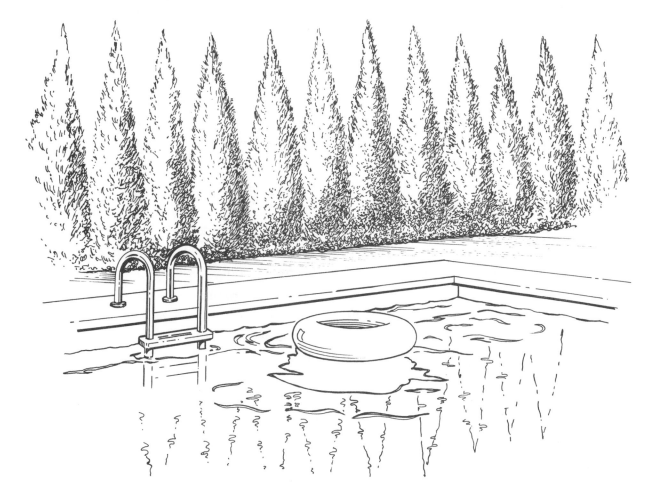

A windbreak around your pool or spa will reduce evaporation and keep the water warmer. A grove of trees, a fence, and an L-shaped corner of a house make good windbreaks.

TEN CRUCIAL QUESTIONS TO ASK BEFORE CONTRACTING WITH A POOL BUILDER

A swimming pool, especially an in-ground pool, is a major purchase. You'll have many options to consider and decisions to make. Happily, you don't have to go it alone. The right pool builder should be able to walk you through design and construction, minimizing headaches and stress levels.

When choosing a pool builder, look for someone who is trustworthy, professional, organized, and communicative. Though delays may occur, sometimes for legitimate reasons, you want to align yourself with a pool builder who can supervise the job from start to finish and keep you apprised of the situation every step of the way. Remember that the research and effort you put in to hiring the right builder will pay off tenfold in the satisfaction you'll have when the job is finally finished.

1. How long has the builder been in business? You want a builder who's experienced and who you can expect will be around for many years, so that he or she can help you with any of your future service needs.

2. Is the builder a licensed contractor? Most states require contractors to be licensed.

3. Does the builder have any complaints on file with the licensing boards or the Better Business Bureau? If so, how were they handled?

4. Is the builder adequately insured to cover any damage that may occur on your property?

5. Will the builder supply a customer list? Ask for the names and addresses of past and current clients whose pools are at various stages of being built. Visit them all so you can see how projects have held up over time and how well job sites are being managed during construction. Ask about the quality of workmanship and the builder's ability to stay on schedule.

6. Does the builder have the design talent and engineering skills to create the pool you envision? Ask to see any industry design awards he may have won or pictures of some projects he's most proud of.

7. Do you understand each party's obligations under the contract? Some areas of concern include: extra charges for encountering difficult soil conditions, extra charges for upgrading electrical service if needed, responsibility for property damage (including sidewalks and driveways), responsibility for replacing lawns and landscaping, consequences of going beyond the agreed-upon schedule, a payment schedule that coincides with the costs incurred during construction, clearly written warranties from the builder and manufacturers of individual components, and responsibility for starting up the pool.

8. Does the builder provide "pool schools" and other training opportunities where you can learn how to maintain your pool?

9. Does the builder service the pools he builds or does he subcontract the service out to another company? Subcontractors may be less responsive than the original pool builder.

10. Do you get a good vibe from the builder? That is, do you like the person and do you feel he or she is someone you can work with? You deserve to get the pool you envision, so you want to make sure the builder you hire is focused on meeting the customer's needs.

Choosing the Right Spa

hether it's a quiet soak in a whirlpool bath or a vigorous jet massage in a backyard spa, the soothing effects of hot-water therapy draw most of us like a magnet. The massaging action of the warm water reduces muscle soreness and stiffness and eases the pain of arthritis. The heat causes blood vessels to dilate, which lowers blood pressure. And the buoyancy of the water reduces the workload on your heart and muscles by as much as 20 percent. Spas are also credited for reducing stress, promoting more restful sleep, mimicking the benefits of exercise for people with type-2 diabetes, and ridding the body of toxins by encouraging sweating. Some people have even found regular hot tub use to aid in efforts to reduce weight and cellulite.

As the list of spa benefits continues to grow, so do the styles and options available. Spas, also known as *hot tubs,* have changed dramatically in design since they were first fashioned from California wine vats in the 1970s. Choosing the right spa for you and your family can be a daunting task. You can spend months researching the purchase by surfing the Internet and visiting stores, but in the end you can end up more confused than when you started out.

This chapter aims to lift you from the quagmire of hot tub data and bring some clarity to your purchase decision. We'll discuss each component of the spa and give you the information you need to make a smart buying decision.

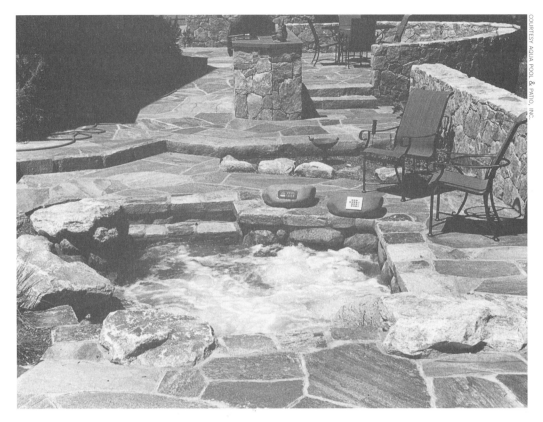

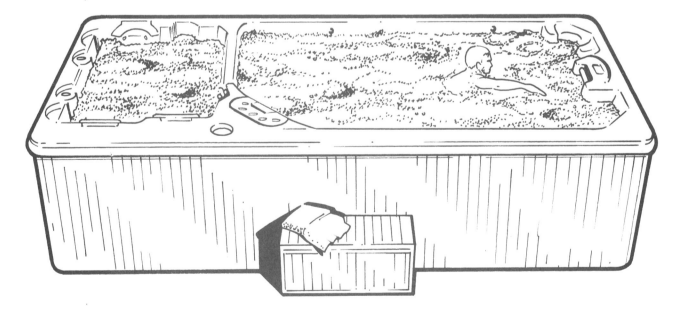 COURTESY AQUA POOL & PATIO, INC.

Custom in-ground spas can be designed and built much like miniature swimming pools. In this spa, the spa-side controls are cleverly hidden within two rocks.

Fitness spas provide warm-water therapy and enough space for an aggressive water workout, making them ideal for small yards or for active people who don't want a full-size pool.

SHELLS

When shopping for a spa, your attention is usually first captured by the shell. A few manufacturers still make traditional hot tubs from wood, but most of today's prefabricated spas are made from acrylic, thermoplastic, fiberglass, tile, or soft vinyl (for those with little space and small budgets). Custom concrete spas are also popular and can be installed alone or in combination with a swimming pool — making their construction more synonymous with concrete pool construction.

Of the shell materials used to create factory-made spas, the most popular is acrylic, because it offers a wide range of color choices, including popular blues and greens, as well as more neutral earth tones that complement most any environment. Acrylic also offers several surface textures, including faux granite and smooth, glossy finishes resembling those of luxury automobiles.

The acrylic sheets used to form spa shells are differentiated by their thickness, the way they're backed for support, and the method used in forming them into spa shells. For example, most spa manufacturers use a single acrylic sheet and reinforce it with a fiberglass backing. Others use an acrylic sheet and a thermoplastic backing that are laminated together.

Just two companies supply the vast majority of acrylic sheeting for spa manufacturing: Ineos Acrylics and Aristech Acrylics. The main difference between the companies' acrylics is color selection. As the companies search for ways to further differentiate their product lines, Ineos has developed an acrylic infused with Microban, a substance that inhibits bacteria growth on the surface. If a spa's water is properly sanitized (see chapter 4), there is no significant health advantage to having a spa shell made with Microban.

Other than color selection, the biggest thing differentiating one spa shell from another is the mold, which determines the seating configuration. A spa can seat anywhere from two to ten or more people, with five or six being the standard occupancy rate. Among these sizes you'll find a variety of seating configurations using myriad combinations of lounges, bucket seats, and benches.

To determine which spa style and size is right for you, think about your lifestyle, home decor, and how you plan to use your new spa. For example, if you're imagining quiet, moonlit soaks with a significant other, a small two-person spa with dual lounges may be sufficient. On the other hand, if you envision wild hot tub parties with a large draw of guests, you'll be drawn to spas with larger seating capacities. And if your spa is going indoors, you'll want to restrict your choices to models that will fit through your doorways. (For more on indoor spa installations, see chapter 3.)

One tip as you go shopping for that perfect spa: Test each spa for comfort by taking off your shoes and sitting in the empty spa on the showroom floor. Better yet, see if you can make an appointment to take a test soak in a fully operational spa. Many spa dealers provide private "mood rooms" for just this purpose. Don't be shy about asking for a test soak. After all, few people would buy a chair without sitting in it first, and a spa purchase is no different.

THE CABINET

Just as visible as the shell is the spa cabinet, or skirt, which encloses the shell and all of the plumbing and equipment. Cabinets have traditionally been made of redwood or cedar, which look beautiful when new but need to be refinished at least annually to maintain their luster. Plus, the wood weakens over time and can break easily, especially if a spa cover removal device is attached to the cabinet, placing extra strain on the wood.

To offer a more durable and maintenance-free cabinet, some manufacturers have begun using simulated wood made from polymers. An embossed wood grain and warm coloring give some of these faux wood cabinets a natural appearance.

Meanwhile, a few spa models eliminate the wood entirely and use the shell material to make the cabinet as well. A cabinet that matches the shell can give a uniform appearance to the spa installation and is a nice option if you don't like the wood designs.

JETS

While the spa shell and cabinet are important for reasons of aesthetics and comfort, the jets merit at least equal attention, because they provide the hydrotherapy effect every spa buyer seeks. Jets have the power to transform a stagnant vessel of water into an aquatic paradise designed for total body relaxation, stress relief, and physical therapy.

A few things to consider about jets:

~ Don't choose quantity over quality. A few well-placed jets that provide just the right hydrotherapy for your body are worth more than dozens of jets that hit you in all the wrong places.
~ Wet-test a spa to make sure the jets are positioned where you'd like them. Most spas are equipped with an *aerator* (air blower) that allows you to control the amount of air introduced into the water streaming from the jets. The introduction of air creates a more intense jet action.

Experiment with the blower options when testing out a spa, especially if you think the jet action is too weak or too strong.

~ Jets come in many styles, including neck jets, stationary jets, cluster jets, oscillating or rotating jets, directional jets, and handheld jets. If the spa you fancy doesn't have a jet configuration that meets your needs, you might be able to have the jets specially placed to suit your specifications.

With the right jet configuration, you'll never want to get out of your hot tub. With the wrong jet configuration, even a comfortable, ergonomically styled seat won't give you a satisfactory hydromassage. On the other hand, if a seat has been properly jetted but is not ergonomically designed, you still won't have a relaxing experience. So shop wisely.

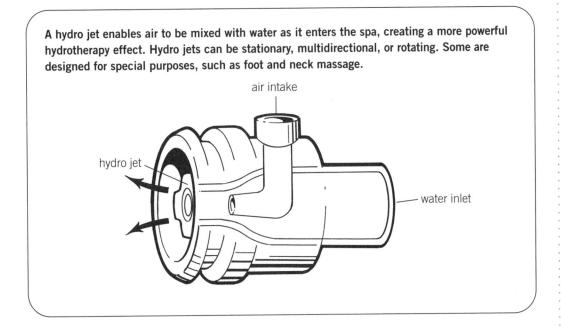

A hydro jet enables air to be mixed with water as it enters the spa, creating a more powerful hydrotherapy effect. Hydro jets can be stationary, multidirectional, or rotating. Some are designed for special purposes, such as foot and neck massage.

air intake

hydro jet

water inlet

PUMPS

Bigger is not better when it comes to spa pumps. Truth be told, an oversized pump can wreak havoc on a spa's plumbing system, as well as waste energy. With a portable spa, the manufacturer has already sized the pump inside the cabinet to work at maximum efficiency for that particular spa model. Trouble can arise, however, when a pump needs to be replaced and the spa owner thinks he or she will get a bigger pump to increase the power of the jets.

Please note that pump sizes can be rated either by their start-up horsepower or by their continuous operating horsepower. When replacing a pump, make sure the new one is rated by the same gauge as the old one was. Also note the number of pumps your spa has and to which tasks each pump is assigned. For example, some units have a two-speed pump — the low speed is used for mild jet action and for circulating the water during the filtration cycles, and the high speed is for greater hydrotherapy. Other spas have a separate 24-hour circulation pump that routes the water through the filter and the heater, thereby allowing the main pump to focus on the single task of providing jet action.

Also, some pumps operate more quietly than others. If you don't want to be shouting to your spa mate during a romantic dip, make sure your spa pump is designed for quiet operation.

For more information on pumps and motors, see chapter 8.

HEATERS

Portable spa heaters are electric and come in two types. One type uses an immersion-style heating element that is placed in direct contact with the water. The other wraps the heating element around a stainless-steel tube through which the water flows.

Immersion-style heaters are more efficient because all of their heat is transferred to the water. However, immersion-style heating elements are apt to deteriorate because of the water's corrosive tendencies. Over time, such heaters can fail, especially if the water is unbalanced. Clearly, the best thing you can do to prolong an immersion-style heater's life is to keep your spa water properly balanced. This prevents the water from becoming overly corrosive.

With a wraparound heating element, not all the heat produced is transferred via the stainless-steel tube to the water, making it less efficient. In fact, only about 60 percent of the heat generated is transferred to the water, compared with 100 percent for immersion-style heaters. However, because the water doesn't come in contact with the heating element, the wraparound-style heater tends to last longer. With greater longevity also comes a higher price tag.

Spa heaters are designed to heat the water to a maximum recommended temperature of 104°F (40°C). Temperatures greater than this may cause bathers to pass out. Most people find a temperature range of 100 to 103°F (38–39°C) to be most comfortable.

Most spa heaters have a 5- to 6-kilowatt capacity, which should be enough to maintain the desired spa temperature, even with the insulating cover removed. However, if you live in a colder climate, check with the spa dealer to make sure the heater for the spa you're considering is powerful enough to heat the water during the winter months. If you're buying a portable spa, which has a self-contained equipment pack, the heater has already been sized correctly. If you're building a custom spa, however, check out the heater sizing information in chapter 9.

FILTERS

The filter screens fine particles and debris out of the spa water. Concrete spas built in conjunction with swimming pools often share the pool's filtration system. Prefabricated stand-alone spas typically use *cartridge filters,* cylinders of pleated fabric held together by end caps. Some spas use one large cartridge filter; others call for several smaller ones.

Cartridge filters should be cleaned every few months or whenever the flow rate of water seems restricted. Cleaning is simply a matter of removing the cartridge and hosing it off with a garden hose, being sure to focus on the deep recesses of the pleats, where dirt accumulates.

If maintained properly, a spa cartridge filter can last one to three years, depending on bather load. When it's time to replace the cartridge filter, be aware that sizing a filter to your particular spa is important. If there is too much pumping action for the filter to handle, unfiltered water can be forced back into the spa. If there isn't enough pumping action to force water through the filter medium, the jet action can be reduced. You spa owner's manual should tell you which size and style of filter is right for your spa. See chapter 7 for more information.

SANITIZING UNITS

Many spas are equipped with sanitizing units that prolong and amplify the effectiveness of the chemical treatment (usually bromine) used to sanitize spa water. In effect, they reduce the amount of sanitizing chemicals you'll need to add to your spa.

The most common spa sanitizing units are ozonators and mineral purifiers. For more information about both, and to learn how to sanitize your spa's water, turn to chapter 4.

CONTROLS

Spa controls allow you to monitor your spa operation from the comfort of the spa or the convenience of your home. They're not complicated; if you can work a microwave oven, you should have no problem figuring out today's spa controls.

Spa controls are an integral part of a prefabricated spa, and you won't have any choice in which one the manufacturer uses. With a custom spa, however, you may get to choose your controls yourself. Either way, test out the controls to make sure their operation makes sense to you. Typically they'll enable you to set the water temperature, turn on and off lights, power up the pumps and blower, see whether the ozonator is operating, and lock the controls so no one can change the temperature or operate the pump while you're away. Some will require you to program the time and duration of your filtration cycles, while others are preprogrammed with this information.

Handheld remote controls are growing in popularity, especially for custom-built spas, and more owners are opting to install control panels in their homes so they don't have to trek out to the spa to check the water temperature, fire up the jets, or turn on the lights. Many spa controls are accessible via telephone, so you can turn on the heater while you're stuck in rush-hour traffic. Future plans for spa controls envision an interface with Web browsers so you could monitor your hot tub from even greater distances. Just imagine being able to check in on your spa throughout the week even if it's located at a vacation home you visit only on weekends.

For more information on spa automation, see chapter 11.

ENERGY CONSUMPTION

Energy conservation continues to be of great concern for many people these days. With the unpredictability of energy prices in many regions, it's wise to be concerned about the energy your new spa will consume.

How much energy your spa consumes depends on several factors, including:

~ The model and size you select
~ The temperature you want to maintain
~ How frequently you use it
~ The outside temperature
~ The cost of energy in your area

A typical four-person spa costs just $10 to $12 per month to heat, based on $.07/kW hour, a set temperature of 102 to 104°F (39–40°C), and approximately 12 to 15 hours of usage during the month (or about 30 to 45 minutes every other day). One recent industry study shows that the average spa costs about $20 per month to heat. Either way, it's rather affordable.

A spa dealer should be able to help you estimate the energy cost of a particular spa in your area.

Spas have a reputation for being great squanders of energy, but given the technological advances used in manufacturing spa shells and covers today, spas may be much more energy-efficient than you think. Better spas use closed-cell polyurethane foam, the same material used in freezers, for insulation. Covers are also using better forms of insulation and are manufactured to form a tight seal around the spa lip.

You can save energy by reducing the temperature of the spa water during nonuse times, shortening the filtration cycles (unless the water is cloudy), and installing the spa in a sheltered area away from wind.

BELLS AND WHISTLES

Some manufacturers design spas that are so enjoyable, luxurious, and pampering that you'll never want to get out of the water. Not so long ago, the hottest spa amenity was lighting. Manufacturers incorporated fiber-optic lighting around the spa lip and underwater lighting that changed color. Built-in cup holders and ice buckets elicited oohs and ahhs from consumers. Now it takes much more. The latest adult toys to hit the spa market are built-in CD/stereo systems and TV screens with waterproof speakers. At least one manufacturer even incorporates Internet access so you can surf the Web while soaking in the hot tub.

Though these bells and whistles are fun to consider, be careful that you don't spend a lot of money on something you won't use a lot. Physical comfort and hydrotherapy should be your overriding concerns. The rest is just frosting on the cake.

SPA INSTALLATIONS

Spa installation can be as simple as placing the unit on a structurally sound deck or as elaborate as recessing it in the ground and surrounding it with stone pavers and lush plantings. The type of installation you choose depends on the type of spa environment you want to create and the size of your budget.

Before settling on an installation site, however, consider whether there's adequate access for your spa to reach the installation site. Is the pathway wide and tall enough? Are there any obstacles that need to be moved? Should any tree branches be cut back? Are gates wide enough for the spa to fit through? In some instances, it may be necessary to use a crane to lift a spa over the house and lower it into place in the backyard. Most professional dealers are prepared for this, and the cost to you should be no more than a few hundred dollars, depending on how far the crane must travel.

That said, here's a brief description of the most popular types of spa installations for you to consider.

In-Ground Installations

Concrete in-ground spas can be installed independently from or in conjunction with in-ground pools. Many spa and pool combinations feature an elevated spa that spills into the pool, thereby creating a water feature that's both inviting to look at and soothing to listen to. These spas are usually surfaced with the same material — plaster, stone aggregate, tile, et cetera — used in the pool.

Some homeowners, however, opt to install prefabricated acrylic or fiberglass spas alongside their concrete pools because of the better seating configurations and hydrotherapy they offer. If your prefabricated spa is being installed below grade, your builder will create a vault, often lined with concrete, to hold your tub. A sump pump or draining system should be included in the vault if there's a possibility of water accumulating in the vault and coming in contact with the spa's electrical equipment.

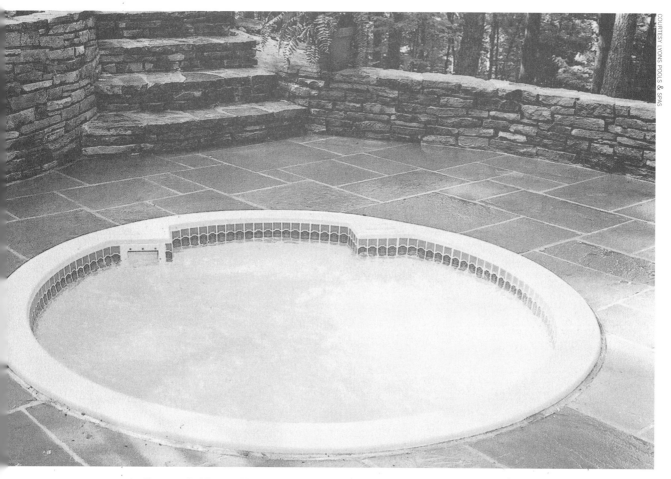

Surrounded by cut bluestone pavers and shaded by a canopy of trees, this in-ground fiberglass spa is a welcome retreat, day or night.

Deck Installations

Wooden decks are a popular location for spas because they provide easy access to and from the home. Before you place a spa on your deck, however, make sure it can support the weight of the spa (including that of the water and a maximum number of bathers). The weight of the spa, when full, is usually supplied in the owner's manual. You'll have to estimate the weight of bathers on your own. Once you know the maximum weight to expect, check with a building contractor or engineer to see if your deck can handle the load. You may need to add structural support beneath the deck area where you plan to set the spa. If you're building a new deck, give your calculations to the deck builder so he or she can design a deck that suits your needs.

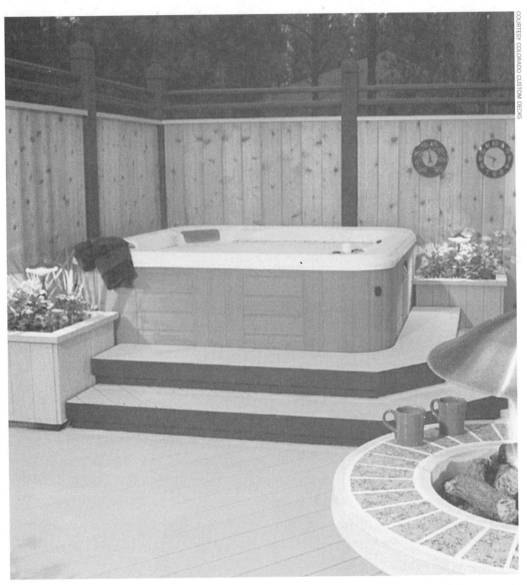

COURTESY COLORADO CUSTOM DECKS

A privacy screen creates an outdoor room for this cozy spa installation with wraparound steps, mood lighting, and gas-fueled fire pit.

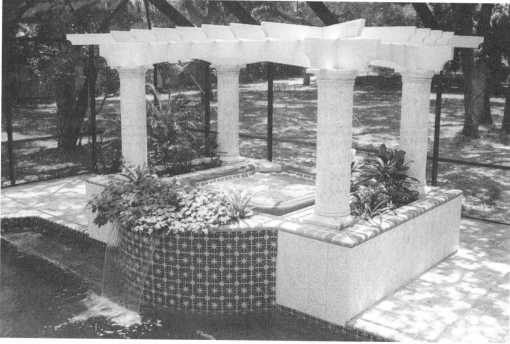

This inviting spa is actually a self-contained unit installed on top of the pool deck, with the arbor built around three of its sides. The design makes it appear as if the spa is spilling into the pool.

Patio Installations

If your spa is being placed on the ground, it must sit on a level, solid foundation. Otherwise, the spa could become damaged, and most warranties are void if the product isn't installed properly. One of the best foundations is a reinforced concrete pad at least 4 inches (10 cm) thick. Some other materials you might be able to use to create a solid foundation are bricks and railroad ties. Just make sure that the surface is stable and won't sink in spots, which could cause the spa to become unleveled.

Indoor Installations

Before placing a spa indoors, make sure that the floor is structurally sound and can support the weight of the spa plus the weight of the water and the bathers. Keep in mind that water will accumulate around the tub, so the floor coverings should be nonslippery and a floor drain should be installed. Steam from the spa will cause water to get into unprotected woodwork and may produce dry rot, mildew, mold, and other problems. Check with an architect to ensure that the room has enough ventilation to prevent moisture damage. (For more information, see chapter 3.)

AQUATIC EXERCISE

One of the best fitness activities is aquatic exercise. It's especially beneficial for those who are overweight or have weak joints, because the buoyancy factor reduces the impact and stress of a workout.

An estimated 6 million people take part in some form of aquatic exercise other than swimming, and much of this exercise is done in warm-water spas. In fact, rehabilitation centers have long used aquatic therapy to speed the recovery process after surgery, and for many years the Arthritis Foundation has promoted a warm-water aquatic exercise program. "Water is a safe, ideal environment for relieving arthritis pain and stiffness," the organization says. "Water exercise is especially good for people with arthritis because it allows you to exercise without putting excess strain on your joints and muscles."

To take advantage of aquatic exercise in the comfort of your own home, you may want to consider a swim spa or fitness spa. Swim spas are large, deep spas with a swim jet on one end that creates a continuous current for users to swim against (see illustration on page 24). Fitness spas have a swim jet but also incorporate various exercise stations for stretching and strength training. And when you're finished with your workout, you can relax in the spa's bench seating, which includes hydrotherapy jets. Like traditional spas, swim and fitness spas use insulating covers to retain heat when no one is using them.

As the trend toward aquatic exercise continues, so does the variety of related products and accessories. These items can be used in a pool or a spa to help you customize an aquatic workout program that's right for you. Most of these products are available through pool and spa supply retailers, on-line retailers, and catalogers.

○ Aqua gloves, which have webbing between the fingers for greater resistance

○ Aqua shoes, for better traction when water walking

○ Aqua weights, which attach to your waist, ankles, and wrists for strength training

○ Kickboards, which support the upper body while exercising the legs

○ Balance boards, which enable swimmers to stand, sit, or kneel with their heads out of the water while they perform dynamic movements with the arms, legs, and waist

○ Inflatable collars and pillows, which help swimmers float on their backs while exercising

○ Exercise balls for stretching, resistance training, and improving eye/hand coordination

○ Flotation devices (such as belts and water noodles) for added buoyancy, especially during aqua jogging

○ Resistance devices, such as arm and leg splints, paddles, fins, and resistance bands

○ Underwater steps, for aerobic exercise and strength training

○ Underwater treadmills

○ Floating barbells for strength training

3

Indoor Pools and Spas

ndoor pools and spas are sheer luxury. Regardless of the weather, you can always enjoy a leisurely swim or a relaxing soak. And your indoor pool and spa room can have windows and sliding doors that open to the outside, giving you a pseudo-outdoor pool and spa setting whenever you fancy one.

But don't make the mistake of assuming that an indoor pool and spa are simply an outdoor pool and spa with four walls and a roof. There's nothing simple about it. Though an indoor pool and spa room may look like the rest of the home architecturally, it's quite different when it comes to engineering. The biggest differences can be seen in the areas of heating and ventilation, which can easily cost as much as the pool and spa themselves. But when you consider how quickly moisture and humidity can ruin your investment, you'll be glad you've invested in the proper air-quality control systems.

PROFESSIONAL ADVICE

Building an indoor pool or spa is not something to undertake on your own. An investment of this magnitude deserves to be done right, and that means hiring an experienced professional who's well versed in the design, construction, and fine nuances of indoor pools and spas. If the architect or builder you hire isn't knowledgeable about indoor pools and spas, you may end up with an

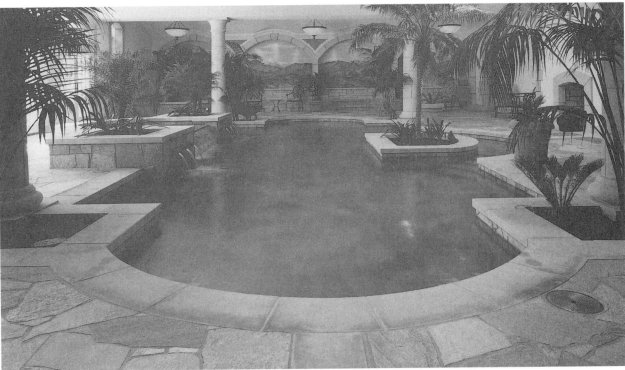

A raised spa and dual water features spill into this elaborate indoor pool, which includes flagstone decking, lush plantings, and a scenic mural. The room also features skylights, a wood-burning fireplace, and a wall of French doors opening to the yard.

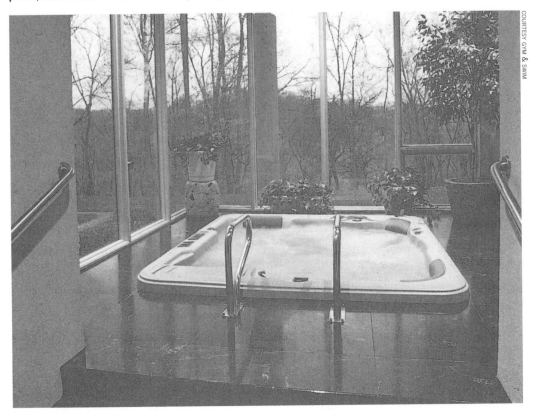

Floor-to-ceiling windows blur the line between indoors and outdoors in this interior spa installation.

area of your home better suited for growing bumper crops of mold and mildew than for hosting festive parties.

Following are some of the areas of greatest concern for indoor pool and spa builders. This brief overview is not intended to help you take on the job yourself. Rather, it will give you the knowledge and confidence necessary to hire the right professional for your project.

EVAPORATION AND HUMIDITY

How much water evaporates from an indoor pool is dependent on five factors:

~ The humidity of the room
~ The surface area of the water
~ The temperature of the water
~ The temperature of the air
~ The number and type of splashing water features

The larger the surface area of the pool or spa, the greater the evaporation. Evaporation also increases when the water is warmer than the air and when the pool contains water features that cause a lot of splashing around. When water evaporates, it causes the water temperature to drop, the air temperature to increase, and the room's humidity level to increase. The resulting warm, moist conditions are nothing short of paradise for molds and mildews, which will thrive in your natatorium to the point of causing structural damage. In short, if there are any costs to be cut, you don't want them to be in the area of air quality. Those who try to skirt around the cost could see ceilings fall and mold and mildew take over. Also, health research has shown that poorly ventilated indoor pool and spa environments can cause respiratory problems if aerosolized water particles carrying bacteria are allowed to enter the lungs.

Your builder or architect will install three types of systems to control evaporation and humidity in your pool and spa room: a dehumidifier, an air-exchange ventilation system, and an insulated pool or spa cover.

Dehumidifiers

To remove evaporated moisture from your pool and spa room, you'll need a dehumidification system that's sized for your particular installation. Most of these systems perform best when the water is 2 to 4 degrees F (1–2 degrees C) warmer than the air. However, if you prefer your pool water to be 10 degrees F (6 degrees C) warmer than the room, or if you have a spa (which typically will be heated to much higher than the room temperature), you'll need a dehumidification system that can handle the corresponding higher rate of evaporation.

To conserve water and energy, you may want a system that diverts water and heat from the dehumidifier back to the pool.

Air-Exchange Ventilation Systems

To maintain healthy air quality, it's important to circulate fresh air through your indoor pool and spa room. An air-exchange system ensures that a fresh supply of air is being brought into the room at all times. It can be part of the dehumidification system; merely exchanging the moist inside air with fresh air from outside will help reduce humidity.

The air-exchange system can also be used to keep windows from fogging up. Maintaining airflow across the entire width of the windows is the only way to keep them clear. For this reason, some architects recommend placing air vents in both the floor and the ceiling near each pane.

An exchange of fresh air will also help keep the pool smell from invading the rest of the home. To quarantine pool-room air in the pool room, your builder will need to make sure that the pool room's ventilation, mechanical, and environmental systems are self-contained and pressurized. This will prevent a gust of pool-house air from blowing into the rest of the house when the adjoining door is opened.

Though modern ventilation systems are capable of reducing chemical odors, there are additional remedies. One is to use less odorous forms of sanitation, such as ozonators and mineral purifiers, which are discussed in chapter 4.

Pool and Spa Covers

Covering up your pool and spa when they're not in use will greatly reduce evaporation and give your dehumidification system a break. For spas, of course, a cover is a necessity for retaining heat and conserving energy. Covers also provide a degree of safety if the pool and spa room is ever accessible by unsupervised children.

For more information about pool and spa covers, see chapter 10.

VAPOR BARRIERS

Vapor barriers — usually thick sheets of overlapping plastic that separate the structural framework and insulation from the drywall — are necessary behind all walls to prevent moisture from reaching the structural framework, where it can foster mold and cause freeze/thaw damage. For the walls themselves, some builders believe that greenboard — a water-resistant drywall often used in bathrooms — is sufficient in pool and spa rooms. Others recommend a waterproof board, such as Wonder Board. Still others recommend Dryvit, a material designed for exterior applications; it's available in several textures and can be painted. Your builder can help you decide which wall material is best for your particular application.

DRAINAGE

Whereas outdoor pools are designed so that water on the surrounding deck drains away from the pool (which keeps debris and lawn chemicals from entering the pool), indoor pools should be planned so that deck water drains *into* either the pool or the deck drains. Otherwise, you risk water damage to the room's structure and the air ducts, which are usually placed around the perimeter of the room. Though some builders don't use deck drains, they can be useful, especially if you're going to be washing the deck with detergents that you don't want to rinse into the pool. Even a simple indoor portable spa, sans pool, should be accompanied by a floor drain. The floor drain is handy when it comes time to drain the spa, and it also sucks down any water splashed out of the spa.

LIGHTING

As much as possible, incorporate natural lighting into your indoor pool and spa room. Copious amounts of skylights and floor-to-ceiling windows help create an outdoor feeling; they make the room feel bright, welcoming, and open. Natural light also enables you to grow real plants in your pool and spa room, further enhancing the outdoor feel.

For nighttime enjoyment, use wall sconces, recessed fixtures in soffits around the room's perimeter, and underwater lights to set the mood and provide a safe swimming environment. Avoid installing light fixtures directly above the pool or spa, because the bulbs — which will eventually need to be changed — are difficult to access, and if they break, you'll surely end up with glass in the water. If you want lighting in the ceiling above the water, install fiber-optic cable fixtures, which use remote illuminators.

HEATING

Indoor pools and spas are heated in the same way as outdoor ones (see chapter 9 for more information). Heating the room itself is another matter. Forced-air

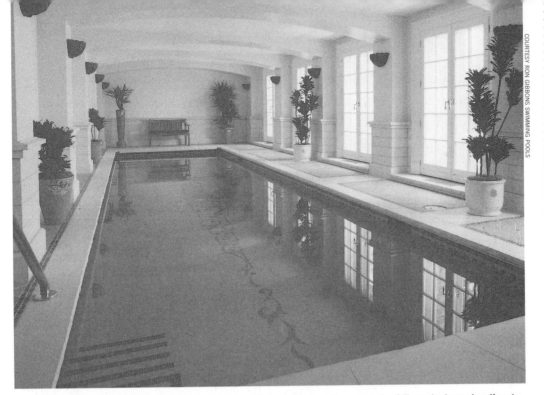

This tiled indoor pool features a decorative motif down the center, a bank of French doors leading to the yard, and wall sconces to illuminate the ceiling for nighttime enjoyment.

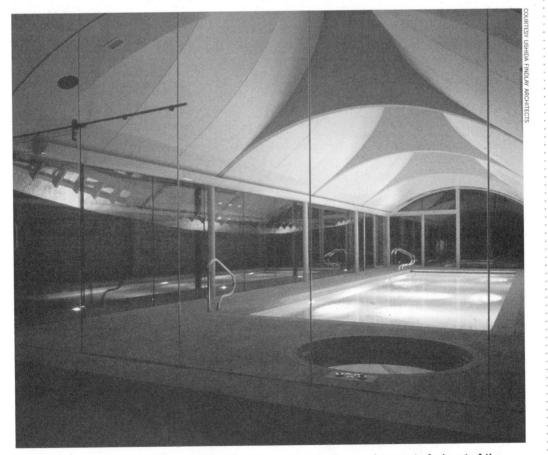

A glass-walled pool house with a skylight along the roof peak allows swimmers to feel part of the surrounding gardens and country landscape.

heat that uses the same ductwork as your air-exchange/dehumidification system is the most common, but it often isn't enough to take the chill out of stone and tile decks. For this reason, some homeowners have in-floor radiant heating systems installed during the pool construction process. Your builder or architect should be able to advise you as to whether such a system would benefit you.

EQUIPMENT ROOM

The equipment room for your indoor pool should be large enough to hold comfortably all the necessary equipment — pumps, filters, automatic sanitizers, heaters, and ventilation equipment — and to provide enough room for service technicians to work on the equipment as needed. Homeowners often want to make the equipment room as small as possible in order to maximize their living space, but a cramped equipment room can lead to problems down the road. If you're working with an architect, make sure he or she is in close communication with the pool builder and that they're discussing the needs and size of the equipment room.

Ideally, the equipment room should have its own entrance, separate from that of the house, so that service technicians can access the equipment without having to walk through the house. Also, every equipment room should have a floor drain.

FINE DESIGN

We've discussed why outdoor pools should be designed for maximum aesthetic value. Your indoor pool should be treated no differently. Indeed, it's increasingly common for indoor pools and spas to be extensions of larger entertainment areas or designed to be viewed through windows from other parts of the home.

In your design of a pool and spa room, don't overlook the possibility of installing adjacent facilities. A changing room, steam room, sauna, and exercise room can all lend to the home health spa and resort atmosphere you're trying to create.

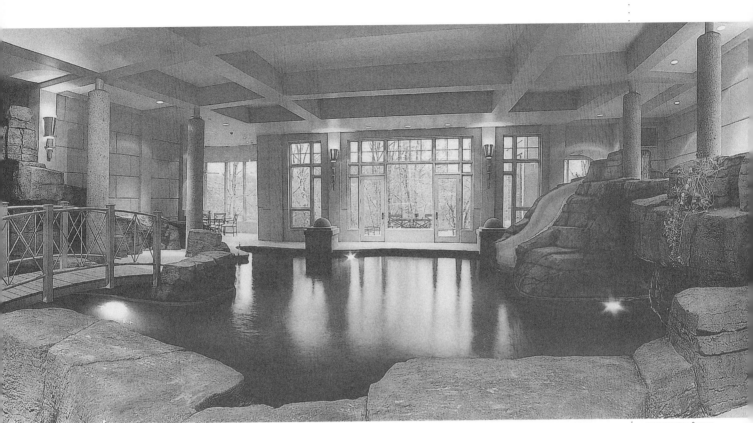

An indoor slide and ceiling-high waterfall add drama and excitement to this indoor pool installation.

Water Chemistry and Testing

As a pool or spa owner, your primary task is to balance the water and maintain proper sanitizer levels, thereby ensuring a safe swimming or soaking environment. To do this, you need some basic knowledge of water chemistry and a familiarity with the various types of sanitizers available for use in pools and spas. If you're diligent about testing the water and adding the proper amounts of the required chemicals, you'll be rewarded with clean, healthy water. If not, you could encounter a host of problems, including algae growth, staining, and corrosive water that damages your investment.

You could, of course, hire a service company to manage the routine care of your pool or spa. However, do-it-yourself maintenance will not only save you money but also provide you with the peace of mind that comes with knowing exactly how clean and safe your water is at all times.

For those who like to know the why behind the how of pool-water chemistry, this chapter is for you. In less time than it takes to blow up a beach ball, you'll know what it means to balance your pool and spa water and how to keep it sparkling clean.

Keep in mind that there is no precise water-treatment method for every pool and spa. Rather, there are guidelines, parameters, and recommendations. Ultimately, it's up to you to determine which method of water treatment you prefer.

FIVE FICKLE FACTORS

Your top priority as a pool or spa owner is to keep the water sanitized. For any sanitizer to work well, however, the water must be balanced. Balanced water is neither corrosive (acidic) nor scale producing (alkaline). Five factors affect water balance: pH, total alkalinity, calcium hardness, total dissolved solids (TDS), and temperature. If any of the five factors is on the low side, metal corrosion, plaster etching, and staining may result. If any are on the high side, you may see cloudy water, staining, and mineral deposits. And in either case, swimmers or soakers will likely experience eye and skin irritation.

A change in any one factor can affect the others, so your challenge is to "balance" the water using various types of chemicals that keep each factor in its proper range. The process may sound complicated, but it isn't as difficult as you think. It just requires a little study on your part so that you understand how each factor contributes to overall water quality and how to adjust it if it's out of whack.

pH

Water pH is a measure of acidity or alkalinity. The pH scale runs from 0 to14, with 7 being neutral. Lower values are acidic, and higher values are alkaline. The acceptable range for pool and spa water is 7.2 to 7.8, though the ideal range is 7.4 to 7.6. Not coincidentally, this is the same pH as that of human eyes — one reason why a proper pH level is important for swimmer or bather comfort.

A low pH means that the water is acidic, also called corrosive. Acidic water can etch metals and plaster, stain plaster finishes, and cause bather discomfort, such as skin and eye irritation. Low pH also causes chlorine sanitizers to dissipate quickly.

When the pH is high, the water is alkaline, also called *scale producing*. Alkaline water can be cloudy and form scale deposits on the pool surface and equipment. As with low pH, high pH levels cause chlorine to become less effective, and skin and eye irritation may occur.

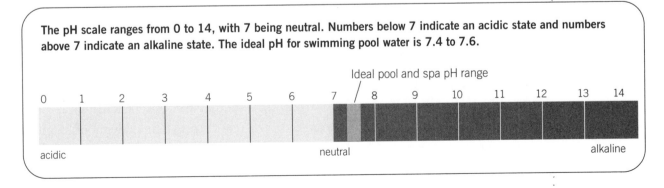

The pH scale ranges from 0 to 14, with 7 being neutral. Numbers below 7 indicate an acidic state and numbers above 7 indicate an alkaline state. The ideal pH for swimming pool water is 7.4 to 7.6.

Ideal pool and spa pH range

0   1   2   3   4   5   6   7   8   9   10   11   12   13   14

acidic   neutral   alkaline

Testing pH. Use test strips or a liquid test kit, available at pool and spa supply stores, to monitor pH levels. Be sure to follow the testing procedures precisely as outlined by the manufacturer.

Adjusting pH. Adding an alkali — such as soda ash (sodium carbonate) — to the water will cause the pH value to rise. Adding an acid — such as muriatic acid or sodium bisulfate — to the water will cause the pH value to fall. The pH can also be adjusted through the use of specially designed products, typically sold with names like pH Up and pH Down, that are available from swimming pool and spa supply retailers. Follow the instructions on the product label when adding any of these pH-altering products.

Keep in mind that most chemicals you'll add to your swimming pool or spa — even those not used for pH control — are acidic or alkaline and therefore will affect the pH level.

If water testing ever becomes confusing or problematic, don't hesitate to call a professional pool service technician to perform the tests for you, or bring a water sample to your pool supply dealer for free testing.

Total Alkalinity

Total alkalinity is the sum of all the alkaline substances in the water. The acceptable range for total alkalinity depends on the sanitizer you use. For example, the ideal range for total alkalinity when using stabilized chlorine, chlorine gas, or bromine as your sanitizer is 100 to 120 parts per million (ppm). The ideal range when using unstabilized chlorine is 80 to 100 ppm. Check the product label or ask a pool specialist for the acceptable total alkalinity range for the sanitizer you're using.

One of the miracles of a proper total alkalinity level is that it can help lock in (or stabilize) the pH level. In other words, once you have total alkalinity in check, pH will tend to remain constant. On the other hand, if the total alkalinity level is too low, pH will fluctuate drastically, making it a constant struggle to maintain perfect water balance.

Testing total alkalinity. Use test strips or a liquid test kit available from pool and spa suppliers to monitor total alkalinity levels. Be sure to follow the testing procedures precisely as outlined by the manufacturer.

Adjusting total alkalinity. To raise total alkalinity without raising pH significantly, add sodium bicarbonate to the water. If you also want to raise pH, use sodium carbonate, a coarse form of baking soda, to raise total alkalinity.

If your source water is extremely *hard* (containing high levels of calcium and magnesium), it's possible that your total alkalinity levels may be too high. Hard water is not necessarily a problem if pH can be brought into the acceptable range and the water remains clear. Use a pH decreaser or liquid muriatic acid to reduce total alkalinity.

Calcium Hardness

Calcium hardness is a measure of the water's calcium content and, therefore, relates to the water's scaling or corrosive tendencies. Too much calcium in the water causes it to precipitate out of the water and leads to deposits on surfaces and piping, while too little leads to plaster, concrete, and grout damage.

The ideal range for calcium hardness is 200 to 400 ppm for pools and 150 to 250 ppm for spas, though some manufacturers recommend a narrower range depending on the type of pool or spa surface you have.

Testing calcium hardness. Use a liquid test kit, available from pool and spa suppliers, to monitor calcium hardness levels. Be sure to follow the testing procedures precisely as outlined by the manufacturer.

Adjusting calcium hardness. Low calcium hardness tends to be a more common problem than high calcium hardness. To raise calcium hardness, carefully add predissolved calcium chloride. In the rare instance that calcium hardness is too high, replace some of the pool or spa water with fresh water.

Total Dissolved Solids

The term *total dissolved solids* (TDS) refers to the concentration of conductive chemicals, bather waste, and other solids that can accumulate in the water, particularly when the water evaporates. You cannot see these solids because they are dissolved in the water, but this does not stop them from corroding metal parts (such as pumps, pipes, and filters). High TDS also reduces sanitizer efficiency and can even make water taste salty. TDS should never be allowed to exceed 1,500 ppm over the start-up TDS level.

TDS is more of a concern for spas than pools because spas have higher temperatures, which lead to greater evaporation and higher concentrations of dissolved solids. Plus, the bather load is heavier in a spa than a pool, meaning that more solids are being introduced to the water via sweat, body oil, soap, shampoo, sunscreen, and, yes, even urine.

Testing TDS. TDS can be tested only with a liquid test kit designed for professional use. If high TDS is a concern for you and your pool isn't being maintained by a professional pool service technician, take a water sample to a pool and spa supply store for professional testing.

Adjusting TDS. The simplest way to lower TDS is to replace some of the pool water with fresh water. Even if the source water is hard (lots of dissolved solids), it will still contain fewer dissolved solids than the water in your pool. For stand-alone spas, it's easiest just to replace the entire volume of water.

CALCULATING THE VOLUME OF YOUR POOL

The different chemicals used to balance pool and spa water are added to the water in amounts determined by the total gallons or liters of water being treated. Therefore, before you can begin to balance your pool or spa water, you need to know how much water your pool or spa holds.

The volume of water in a spa is usually noted in the manufacturer's owner's manual, but if you own a pool, you may need to calculate its volume on your own. Here's how to calculate the approximate number of gallons in various pool shapes. (To convert gallons to liters, simply multiply the number of gallons by 3.7854.)

Circular Pools

For pools with straight sides — like aboveground pools — first determine the radius, which is half the diameter, in feet. Then square the radius (or in other words, multiply it by itself). Multiply this number by 3.14 (the value of pi), and then again by the pool's average depth in feet. Finally, multiply by 7.5 (the number of gallons in a cubic foot).

Example
Diameter = 24, so radius = 12
12 x 12 = 144
144 x 3.14 = 452
452 x 4 = 1,808
1,808 x 7.5 = 13,560 gallons (51,330 L)

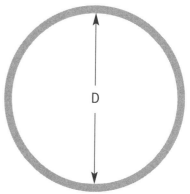

Rectangular Pools

Multiply the length by the width, then multiply by the average depth in feet. Finally, multiply by 7.5.

Example
40 x 28 = 1,120
1,120 x 5 = 5,600
5,600 x 7.5 = 42,000 gallons (158,987 L)

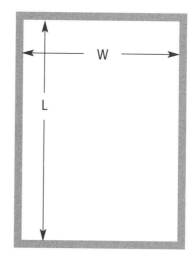

Oval Pools

For pools with straight sides, break the shape into a circle and a rectangle, using the two ends for the circle and the center section for the rectangle. Then calculate the volume of each using the formulas above and add the two numbers together to determine the total volume.

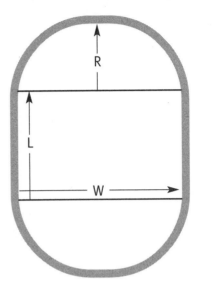

Example
Circle
Diameter = 28, so radius = 14
14 x 14 = 196
196 x 3.14 = 615
615 x 3 = 1,845
1,845 x 7.5 = 13,838 gallons (52,382 L)

Rectangle
32 x 28 = 896
896 x 4.5 = 4,032
4,032 x 7.5 = 30,240 gallons (114,470 L)

Volume of Circle + Volume of Rectangle = 44,078 gallons (166,852 L)

Irregular Pools

Try dividing the pool into smaller shapes that resemble circles, ovals, and rectangles. Calculate the volume of the individual areas, then add the totals. An L-shaped pool, for example, is really just two rectangles; calculate the volume of each and add the two to find the volume of the whole.

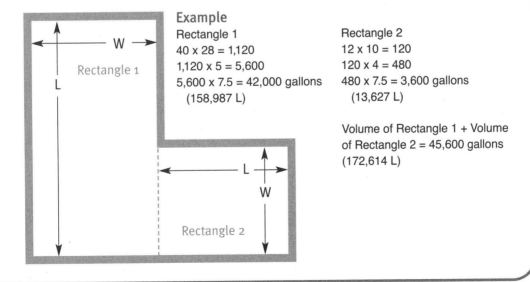

Example
Rectangle 1
40 x 28 = 1,120
1,120 x 5 = 5,600
5,600 x 7.5 = 42,000 gallons
   (158,987 L)

Rectangle 2
12 x 10 = 120
120 x 4 = 480
480 x 7.5 = 3,600 gallons
   (13,627 L)

Volume of Rectangle 1 + Volume of Rectangle 2 = 45,600 gallons (172,614 L)

Temperature

The ideal temperature for pool water is 78 to 82°F (26–28°C). For spas, the temperature should not exceed 104°F (40°C).

Temperature can have a significant effect on water balance because calcium becomes less soluble as water temperature increases and more soluble as the temperature decreases. Said another way, warm water tends to be more scale producing, while colder water tends to be more corrosive. With a spa, where the water temperature is consistently over 100°F (38°C), calcium easily becomes less soluble and needs to be kept in check by closely monitoring the other water-balance factors. Temperature plays a lesser role in pools, but if your pool is being kept at a high temperature, you may need to adjust one or more of the other four factors to compensate.

Pool and spa thermometers, which usually are kept tethered to a handrail or other fixture and dangling in the water, are available at pool and spa supply stores. Electronic thermometers can also relay temperature readings to in-home control panels. Most spas have a built-in thermostat that transmits the temperature to a convenient spa-side display.

The Saturation Index

Maintaining perfect water-balance can be tricky at times. Fortunately, a mathematical formula can help you understand the intricate relationship among all of the water-balance factors. Called the Saturation Index, it was derived from the work of Wilfred F. Langelier, who was commissioned in the 1930s to discover a method for laying down a thin layer of scale on the water-distribution piping of a large city to protect the cast-iron pipes from corrosion. Applied to the pool and spa industry, the index looks like this:

SI = pH + TF + CH + ALK – CONSTANT

SI = saturation index

pH = measured pH

TF = temperature factor

CH = measured calcium hardness

ALK = measured alkalinity minus cyanurate alkalinity, which is the alkalinity attributed to cyanurate acid, used to stabilize pH in swimming pools

CONSTANT = combined factor that corrects for temperature, as well as the strength and concentration of ions in the water

Water is considered balanced when the SI equals 0. An SI of +/–0.3 is considered acceptable. Above 0.3 indicates that conditions are ripe for cloudiness and scaling; below –0.3 points warns of possible corrosive conditions.

This type of advanced mathematics, however, could drive the average pool and spa owner to rethink his or her purchase. Happily, at least one company has produced a simple-to-use tool that does the math for you. Developed by Taylor Technologies, the Watergram is simply two circular charts, one small and one large, laid together and riveted through the center. The smaller inner circle is printed with numbers for pH and calcium hardness, while the outer circle has numbers for total alkalinity and temperature. Let's say you've measured the pH and taken the temperature of your pool. You'd locate that pH reading on the inner wheel and the temperature reading on the outer wheel. When you turn the inner wheel so that the pH reading and the temperature reading are in a line, the wheel will tell you whether total alkalinity or calcium hardness needs to be adjusted.

For more information on the Watergram, visit www.taylortechnolgies.com, where you can also get information on the company's booklet, *Pool & Spa Water Chemistry: A Testing & Treatment Guide*.

SANITIZERS AND OXIDIZERS

Water balance is important, but it's even more crucial to have enough active sanitizer in the water to ensure a safe and healthy swimming or soaking environment. Sanitizers kill pollutants such as algae and bacteria. Oxidizers, in addition to sanitizing, "burn up" or remove accumulated waste products, such as sweat, body oil, shampoo, soap, and urine. Pool and spa water needs both a sanitizer for continual disinfection and an oxidizer for periodic oxidation. Some common sanitizers, such as chlorine and bromine, also oxidize. Others, such as biguanide, are only sanitizers and require a separate oxidizing chemical to work effectively.

Chlorine

Chlorine is the most popular swimming pool sanitizer. It is both a sanitizer and an oxidizer. Different types of chlorine have different effects on the water's pH; you'll need to take this into account when balancing your water and choosing a chlorine product.

One of the drawbacks to chlorine is that it tends to dissipate in sunlight. On a sunny day, for example, it might take as little as two hours for roughly 95 percent of the active

When mixing granular chlorine with water, always add the chlorine to the water, and never vice versa. This helps prevent chlorine from splashing out of the bucket and damaging skin, clothing, and other surfaces.

CAUTION!

chlorine in a pool to be lost. For this reason, chlorine generally needs to be paired with a stabilizing agent, such as cyanuric acid. Of course, some types of chlorine — notably dichlor and trichlor — are more stable in sunlight than others.

Chlorine is also unstable at high temperatures. Therefore, most experts recommend bromine, which is much more stable than chlorine at high temperatures, as a sanitizer for spas.

High pH drastically reduces the effectiveness of chlorine, because it accelerates the rate at which chlorine molecules break down. (The active hypochlorous acid molecule breaks up into an inactive hydrogen ion and a hypochlorite ion.) Pools that run at high pH levels require higher levels of chlorine to kill off algae and bacteria.

After chlorine is no longer able to kill organisms, it combines with contaminants in the pool to form chloramines, nasty little molecules that can irritate eyes and skin and cause a strong chlorinelike odor. In fact, although many people assume that a strong chlorine odor is an indication that there is too much chlorine in the water, actually the opposite is true. The strong odor usually means that the chlorine in the water is no longer an effective sanitizer and chloramines have formed. The solution to this problem is to superchlorinate or "shock" the water (see page 55) with an oxidizer to eliminate the chloramines.

Testing chlorine levels. Use test strips or a test kit (available from pool and spa suppliers) to measure "free available" chlorine — that is, the portion of chlorine that's capable of sanitizing, killing germs, and oxidizing organics. When free available chlorine reacts with ammonia wastes, it becomes "combined chlorine," or, in other words, chloramines. Whereas free chlorine has no detectable taste or smell at levels up to 10 to 20 ppm, combined chlorine levels as low as 0.2 ppm can create the familiar chlorine odor common to heavily used pools. Combined chlorine has few sanitizing capabilities.

For pools, the recommended level of free available chlorine is 2 to 3 ppm. For spas, the recommended level is 3 to 5 ppm. Make sure you're testing for free available chlorine; a reading of total chlorine (free available plus combined chlorine) won't tell you if you have enough active sanitizer in the water.

Adjusting chlorine levels. Chlorine comes in many forms: liquid, granular, tablet, stick, and gas. To add liquid or granular chlorine to the pool, carefully pour it around the pool's perimeter, as far away from the walls as you can reach to help distribute it equally. Some granular formulas do not dissolve quickly, in which case you will want to predissolve them in a bucket of water before adding them to the pool.

To distribute tablet or stick chlorine, place the tablets or sticks in a floating or in-line dispenser. As water flows through the dispenser, the chlorine is dissolved and released gradually.

Chlorine gas should be applied only by a professional.

Figuring "dosage." The different types of chlorine contain different amounts of free available chlorine. The manufacturer of a particular chlorine product should supply a chart that tells you how much chlorine to add to various volumes of water to raise the level of free available chlorine 1 ppm. You may need to do some math to figure out what's appropriate for your specific pool or spa. For example, the package tells you to add X amount to a 5,000-gallon pool and Y amount to a 20,000-gallon pool to increase the chlorine level 1 ppm, then the amount you need to add to a 30,000-gallon pool is X + X + Y (enough for 5,000 + 5,000 + 20,000 = 30,000 gallons).

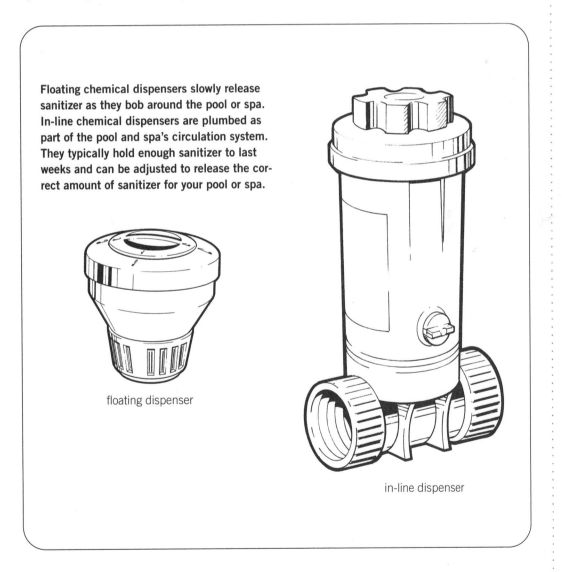

Floating chemical dispensers slowly release sanitizer as they bob around the pool or spa. In-line chemical dispensers are plumbed as part of the pool and spa's circulation system. They typically hold enough sanitizer to last weeks and can be adjusted to release the correct amount of sanitizer for your pool or spa.

floating dispenser

in-line dispenser

Bromine

Like chlorine, bromine is both a sanitizer and an oxidizer. It has little odor, which makes it an enticing product for many pool and spa owners. But unlike chlorine, bromine cannot be stabilized. Thus, just a couple of hours of exposure to sunlight may deplete as much as 65 percent of a bromine residual (the amount of active bromine in the water after the immediate sanitizer demand has been met). Because there is no known way to retain a reliable residual of bromine in sunlight, many experts recommend bromine as a sanitizer only for indoor pools and portable spas, which are usually covered when not in use.

One advantage of bromine, however, is that it can be regenerated. In other words, spent bromine can be reactivated by the addition of, among other chemicals, chlorine. In fact, active chlorine will always regenerate spent bromine before it sanitizes water. So if you're ever thinking about switching your pool or spa's sanitizing system from bromine to chlorine, you'll have to completely drain and refill it so that there's no bromine present.

Testing bromine levels. Test methods for bromine levels are similar to those used for chlorine, except that there's no way to distinguish between combined bromine and free available bromine. Thus, you'll be measuring total bromine residual. The ideal range of bromine residual for residential and spas is 4 to 6 ppm.

Adjusting bromine levels. Bromine is sold as slow-dissolving tablets that are placed in a brominator, which allows water to pass through and provides a steady supply of hypobromous acid to the pool or spa. The fastest way to raise the bromine level is to add a bromine shock, chlorine, or potassium monopersulfate (a nonchlorine oxidizer), all of which will regenerate the bromine bank.

Biguanide

Biguanide was first developed as a pre-surgery antimicrobial scrub. It is the only nonhalogen sanitizer and oxidizer available for pools and spas. (Both chlorine and bromine belong to the halogen family of chemicals.) Some pool and spa owners prefer biguanide because it's less susceptible to UV rays than chlorine and bromine are, doesn't require a stabilizer, doesn't degrade with high temperatures or changes in pH, and usually needs to be applied only every couple of weeks. Also, with biguanide, the water doesn't smell of chlorine, of course, and biguanide reduces the surface tension of the water, which translates to a smoother feel. And at recommended concentrations, biguanide won't irritate the skin or eyes.

Biguanide is not without its faults, however. It has a tendency to gum up filters, sometimes complicating filter cleaning. It also is incompatible with chlorine, bromine, copper-based chemicals, and nonchlorine shock, such as potassium monopersulfate, though it is not at odds with other water-balancing chemicals. Several companies offer complete biguanide pool and spa care systems, which tell you exactly how much of which product to put into the water and when. Follow the instructions carefully and you shouldn't encounter any problems.

Testing biguanide levels. Biguanide levels are monitored with special test kits designed specifically for this purpose. Though biguanides are not new to the world of sanitization, they are the new kid on the block in the world of pools and spas. To ensure proper use, be sure to follow the manufacturer's testing and application guidelines precisely.

Adjusting biguanide levels. Biguanide is available in liquid form; the acronym for its chemical name is PHMB, and you may see these letters on the package label. You'll need to add biguanide to pool and spa water only about every 10 to 14 days, but you should still test the water regularly to make sure it's balanced. Follow the manufacturer's directions carefully to determine how much biguanide to add to your pool or spa and how often. And always check with your biguanide dealer before adding supplemental chemicals to biguanide-sanitized water.

Shock

Shock is a concentrated form of chlorine, potassium monopersulfate, or, less often, bromine that's used to super-sanitize pool and spa water. Shocking burns up bacteria, algae, nitrogen compounds, and smelly ammonia that have not been removed through routine sanitization. Maintaining the proper sanitizer residual will keep your pool water safe for swimming, but shocking the water is sometimes necessary to remove dead bacteria and organic matter that could be causing skin and eye irritations, cloudy water, or foul odors.

The best time to shock your pool or spa is after sundown, which eliminates the dissipating effect of the sun's ultraviolet rays and ensures that the chemical stays in the water at least overnight. After shocking a pool or spa with chlorine, you shouldn't enter the water until the residual has dropped below 10 ppm.

Before shocking, always bring the water-balance factors into the proper range. Otherwise, metals suspended in the water could become insoluble, fall to the bottom, oxidize, and stain the pool or spa surface.

Automatic Sanitizers

If you have a few extra bucks and would prefer the convenience and peace of mind of an automatic pool sanitizer, you have a few options.

Recommended Water Balance for Halogen-Based Sanitizers

POOL/SPA TYPE	COMPONENT	MINIMUM LEVEL	IDEAL LEVEL	MAXIMUM LEVEL
Aboveground or on-ground residential pool	Free chlorine (ppm)	1.0	2.0–4.0	10.0
	Combined chlorine (ppm)	0.0	0.0	0.2
	Bromine (ppm)	2.0	4.0–6.0	10.0
	PHMB (biguanide) (ppm)	30.0	30.0–50.0	50.0
	pH	7.2	7.4–7.6	7.8
	Total alkalinity (ppm as $CaCO_3$)	60	80–100[a]/100–120[b]	180
	Calcium hardness (ppm as $CaCO_3$)	150	200–400	1,000
	Total dissolved solids (ppm)	—	—	1,500 ppm over start-up TDS level
	Temperature	personal preference	78–82°F (26–28°C)	104°F (40°C)
	Ozone (ppm in air above water)	—	—	0.1[c]
In-ground residential pool	Free chlorine (ppm)	1.0	2.0–4.0	10.0
	Combined chlorine (ppm)	0.0	0.0	0.2
	Bromine (ppm)	2.0	4.0–6.0	10.0
	PHMB (biguanide) (ppm)	30.0	30.0–50.0	50.0
	pH	7.2	7.4–7.6	7.8
	Total alkalinity (ppm as $CaCO_3$)	60	80–100[a]/100–120[b]	180
	Calcium hardness (ppm as $CaCO_3$)	150	200–400	1,000
	Total dissolved solids (ppm)	—	—	1,500 ppm over start-up TDS level
	Temperature	personal preference	78–82°F (26–28°C)	104°F (40°C)
	Ozone (in water)	—	—	0.1[c]
Residential spa	Free chlorine (ppm)	2.0	3.0–5.0	10.0
	Combined chlorine (ppm)	0.0	0.0	0.2
	Bromine (ppm)	2.0	4.0–6.0	10.0
	PHMB (biguanide) (ppm)	30.0	30.0–50.0	50.0
	pH	7.2	7.4–7.6	7.8
	Total alkalinity (ppm as $CaCO_3$)	60	80–100[a]/100–120[b]	180
	Calcium hardness (ppm as $CaCO_3$)	100	150–250	800
	Total dissolved solids (ppm)	—	—	1,500 ppm over start-up TDS level
	Temperature	personal preference	personal preference	104°F (40°C)
	Ozone (in water)	—	—	0.1[c]

[a] For calcium hypochlorite, lithium hypochlorite, or sodium hypochlorite
[b] For sodium dichlor, trichlor, chlorine gas, or bromine
[c] Over 8-hour time, weighted average.

Source: Reprinted from National Spa and Pool Institute, *Standard for Residential Swimming Pools*, ANSI/NSPI-5 2003.

Chlorine and bromine generators. These electrical units generate chlorine or bromine from special salts added to the water; some units regenerate a bromine bank already in the water. Chlorine and bromine generators are great for maintaining a sanitizer residual, although periodic shocking is still required.

Ozonators. An ozonator produces and releases ozone — an effective sanitizer — into pool or spa water. However, ozone doesn't last long in a water environment. Once it kills bacteria, the ozone reverts to oxygen and either dissolves into the water or escapes into the air. There's no way to maintain a measurable ozone residual to ensure the water is sanitized as new contaminants are introduced. Therefore, an ozonator must be used in conjunction with small amounts of chlorine or bromine. There are two types of ozonators: UV and corona discharge. A UV unit creates ozone with a special lightbulb, which needs to be replaced after many months. A corona discharge unit has a special cell that produces ozone. Corona discharge ozonators cost more than UV ozonators, but they don't have any bulbs that need replacing.

Ionizers. As water flows through these electrical devices, they introduce silver, copper, and zinc ions into the water. These ions are powerful sanitizers. Like ozone, however, there's no way to maintain a measurable ion residual in the water, so ionizers must be used in conjunction with a halogen-based sanitizer to guarantee a sanitizer residual.

Mineral purifiers. These devices use a combination of silver, copper, and zinc to sanitize water. Some mineral purifiers are simply perforated cylinders that fit inside cartridge filters, whereas others are plumbed in-line along with the other pool equipment. As water flows through a purifier and over the mineral bed, it picks up ions that kill bacteria. Mineral purifiers last several months, but they do not create a sanitizing residual, so they must be used with chlorine or bromine.

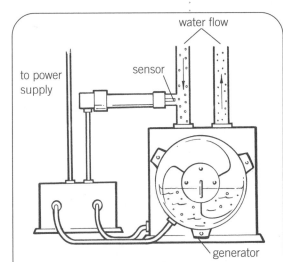

CHLORINE or BROMINE GENERATOR: As water passes through a chlorine or bromine generator, a sensor measures the sanitizer level. If it is low, the unit starts producing more sanitizer from special salts in the water. Once the sanitizer level is in the proper range, the sensor tells the unit to stop producing chlorine or bromine.

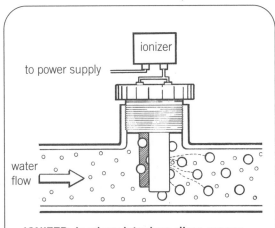

IONIZER: Inonizers introduce silver, copper, and zinc ions into the water to kill bacteria.

ROUTINE CARE

Several chemical manufacturers offer simple step-by-step maintenance programs that tell you which bottle of what to dump into your pool or spa and when to do so. And appendix A outlines the general requirements of routine care for a pool or spa. Stay on schedule and you'll eliminate most of your water worries.

If you're diligent about pool and spa water care, you may never come upon a crisis. If you do, however, don't despair. There's a product designed to combat most any situation you encounter. See chapter 5 for details.

STRICTLY SPAS

Though much of the water-balance and water-treatment information discussed in this chapter applies to both pools and spas, water chemistry for spas entails some unique concerns arising from two factors: the high temperature of the water and the relatively low volume of water per bather.

The water in a typical spa is heated to 98–104°F (37–40°C) — much warmer than the typical 78°F (26°C) swimming pool. High temperatures promote scale formation, evaporation that leads to a high level of total dissolved solids, bacteria growth, high levels of bather waste, and fast chemical reactions.

The small volume of water in a spa means that filtration rates are high (water turns over about once every 25 minutes), bather loads are heavy, sanitizer reserves are low, pH fluctuates easily, and chemical dosing must be more precise. Experts are fond of pointing out that two people in a hot tub create contamination proportionate to that of 60 people in a pool. Another queasy fact: One person in a spa produces about 1 liter of sweat per hour.

Despite the grossness of such factoids, rest assured that hot tub use is safe and healthy if the water is sanitized and balanced per industry standards. Refer to the chart on page 56 for the recommended water-balance parameters for spas.

Spa Chemicals

Regarding spa sanitizers, most experts recommend bromine over chlorine because bromine is more stable at high temperatures. Bromine is available in both granular and tablet form. You can use granular bromine to bring the sanitizer level up to the recommended 4 to 6 ppm quickly, then use tablets in a floating device or chemical feeder to maintain a residual. The number of tablets you'll need will depend on such factors as spa size, frequency and duration of filtration cycles, and bather load.

Always follow the manufacturer's directions carefully when adding chemicals to your spa, and allow the water to circulate for at least 15 minutes before retesting and adding more chemicals. If total dissolved solids is high, simply drain and refill the spa with fresh water; the low volume of water in a spa makes this the most economical solution.

Many spas come equipped with an ozonator. Though ozone is an effective sanitizer, remember that there's no way to maintain or test for a residual of ozone in the water. This means you'll still need to use bromine or chlorine to maintain a measurable sanitizer residual.

You'll also need to shock your spa water almost twice as often as your pool water, or about every week, depending on the bather load.

Draining

Because of heavy bather loads and the constant addition of chemicals, spa water can take on a high concentration of dissolved solids, making the water difficult to balance. To ensure water quality and keep the water easy to balance, most experts recommend draining your spa water at least every three months — more often if the spa is used heavily.

Some experts suggest this formula to determine how often to change the water: spa size in gallons, divided by number of daily bathers times three.

Example

If you have a 500-gallon spa that's used by two people every day:

$500 \div (3 \times 2) = 500 \div 6 = 83$

You should change the water every 83 days, or every two to three months.

Between drainings, you can reduce the contaminants in your spa by having bathers shower before jumping into the tub.

If you do encounter a water problem you can't solve, don't hesitate to bring a water sample to your hot tub dealer and ask for help. Most retailers offer a complete line of problem-solving chemicals, from algaecides and stain removers to scum preventives and defoamers.

10 TIPS FOR ACCURATE WATER TESTING

Balancing pool and spa water becomes a futile task if you don't know how to test the water properly. Everything from improper storage of test kits to timing can cause false readings — and false readings can prompt you to take the wrong course of action.

First, you need to decide which type of testing method you will use. The most accurate results tend to come from liquid test kits. These kits require you to add drops of chemical reagents to a sample of water from your pool or spa and either match the color it yields with those on a comparator chart or count drops needed until the sample changes color.

An easier method is test strips, which typically require you to dip or swirl a strip in the water sample and match the resulting colors on the strip to the corresponding charts on the test strip bottle.

Test strips are available for measuring chlorine levels, bromine levels, pH, and alkalinity. Liquid test kits are available for measuring each of these plus calcium hardness.

Most pool and spa dealers offer free professional water testing; all you have to do is bring in a water sample in a clean container. Many dealers will even print out an analysis that tells you precisely which chemicals, and how much of each, to add to your pool or spa.

That said, you will at some point want or need to test your water on your own at home. To ensure the most accurate results for your analysis, follow these guidelines.

1. Take your water sample from at least 12 to 18 inches (30–45 cm) below the surface. Water near the surface often has a lower sanitizer residual than the rest of the water and can have a higher pH due to evaporation and UV rays near the surface. To get a good sample, invert a clean jar or vial and plunge it up to your elbow beneath the surface of the water. Then upright the jar or vial and fill it.

2. Don't take water samples from near return inlets. If the pool or spa has an in-line chemical feeder, the concentration of sanitizer will be higher there than in the rest of the pool or spa.

3. If your pool has dead spots — areas with poor circulation — test samples taken from several locations.

4. Always use a cap, not your fingers, to seal a test jar or vial. Otherwise, contaminants from your skin can skew pH readings.

5. Perform tests quickly, before the sample has time to change. Exposure to the oxygen in air especially affects chlorine and bromine readings. It is not necessary to cool spa water before testing, either.

6. To get an accurate read on color-based tests, don't wear sunglasses, and perform the test outdoors in natural daylight. Some experts recommend having the sun behind you or using a white piece of paper as a background. Also, hold the test vial at eye level.

7. When squeezing drops of liquid reagents from a bottle, hold the bottle in a vertical position so that the drops are uniform in size.

8. Make sure reagents and test strips are fresh. Experts recommend replacing reagents and test strips annually to ensure freshness. To keep supplies fresh, close reagent and test strip containers as soon as you're finished with them. Make sure your fingers are dry before reaching into a bottle of test strips to keep moisture out. And store supplies in a cool, dry place out of sunlight and away from treatment chemicals.

9. Don't try to substitute reagents from one test kit with another. The color standards, sample sizes, and reagent concentration may differ between kits.

10. Follow the instructions on product labels carefully. If a test calls for the sample to be swirled, don't shake it. If it says "dip," don't swish. Also, watch the clock. Some test strips are designed to be read immediately, while others call for a 30-second waiting period. Waiting too long or reading too soon will not yield an accurate water analysis.

CHEMICAL SAFETY

Like household cleaners and solvents, pool and spa chemicals can be dangerous if handled improperly. They can irritate skin, damage eyes, or even start a fire if stored improperly. Follow these guidelines whenever handling pool and spa chemicals.

- Store sanitizers in a cool, dry place away from other chemicals, out of direct sunlight, and out of the reach of children.

- Do not store liquid chemicals above other chemicals, including garden fertilizers and insecticides, where they could possibly drip and cause a dangerous chemical reaction.

- Wear safety goggles and rubber gloves when mixing and dispensing chemicals.

- Never mix different types of products together.

- If mixing with water is required, never add water to chemicals. Rather, add chemicals to water to eliminate harmful splashing and gassing.

- Use clean, dry plastic cups or scoops for measuring specific products. Never put a wet measuring scoop back in a container.

- Do not inhale fumes or allow products to contact eyes, ears, nose, or mouth.

- Always follow the manufacturer's instructions when dispensing any spa or pool chemical.

- Read the first-aid instructions given on each product's label before using it. Have emergency medical and poison-control-center phone numbers handy at all times.

- Do not smoke when using products.

- Keep products away from lawns and landscaping.

- If a chemical spill occurs, follow the cleanup instructions given on the product label.

5

Common Water Problems

Itchy eyes . . . dry skin . . . faded swimsuits . . . cloudy water . . . plaster bottoms that feel like 100-grit sandpaper — these are just a few of the problems caused by improperly balanced water in your pool or spa. In fact, many pool and spa problems you might think would originate with the filtration system are actually caused by poor water quality. Fortunately, you don't have to be a Nobel Prize–winning chemist to keep your pool and spa water in check.

Routine water tests and the proper application of sanitizers and water-balancing chemicals, as described in chapter 4, will keep your pool or spa water sparkling and safe. But few pool and spa owners have a perfect record of maintenance. Of course, you can always consult a professional service company to take care of any water problem you encounter. But if you're up to the challenge, don't be afraid to tackle these common water worries yourself.

There are a host of chemicals to help you solve most any pool or spa water crisis. If you're ever in doubt about which chemical to use, ask your local pool supply professional. Most pool supply companies offer free water analysis and can prescribe just the remedy you're looking for. In no time, you'll be relaxing in your backyard oasis, enjoying a perfectly balanced and germ-free pool.

ALGAECIDES

Algaecides are used to kill algae and prevent them from taking root in your pool or spa. It's important to make sure the algaecide you use is designed to treat the type of algae you have. Floating green algae are the most common, but there are also yellow/mustard algae and black algae. The product label will tell you which kind of algae it's designed to eliminate.

Algae can grab hold of pool walls and lurk in tight corners where the water doesn't circulate well. After you pour the algaecide into the pool, it may be necessary to brush the area of the algae bloom to make sure that all of the cells are exposed to the algaecide in the water.

CLARIFIERS

Clarifiers herd small particles into clusters large enough to be caught by the pool's filtration system. Sometimes these particle clusters are heavy enough to fall out of solution. Once they settle on the pool bottom, they can be vacuumed up easily. The family of clarifiers includes flocculants, sequestering agents, and chelating agents.

Flocculants are compounds, such as alum, that cause small particles of suspended dirt or other materials to clump together into larger masses so they can be filtered out more easily.

Sequestering agents are chemicals that cause small particles of metals to combine so that they are large enough to be trapped by the filter.

Chelating agents are chemicals that prevent minerals in solution in a body of water from precipitating out of solution and depositing on the surfaces that contain the water.

DEFOAMERS

When certain algaecides are used and/or pH is out of whack, the water begins to foam when agitated. This is especially a problem with spas, which have blowers that introduce air into the water via the jets. For an immediate solution, add a few drops of defoamer to the water and allow them to circulate for several minutes. If the foam remains, repeat the process until the foam is gone.

As a long-term solution to foaming, make sure the water is balanced, shock the water, and/or replace some of the water with fresh water.

SCUM REMOVERS/PREVENTERS

Body oils, lotions, soaps, cosmetics, and other bather waste can accumulate on the water surface and cause unsightly blemishes around the spa and pool waterline. This scum is rarely harmful, but it can be gross. Many over-the-counter tile cleaners will remove scum from spa and pool waterlines, although your pool and spa supply dealer may also recommend some specialty chemicals. To prevent scum from forming, use a scum-absorbing product available from your dealer, and have bathers shower before entering the water.

STAIN REMOVERS

Stains are usually organic (caused by the tannins leaching out of plant debris that makes its way into the water) or metallic (caused by low pH, resulting in corrosive water that attacks the metals found in pool and spa equipment and fittings). Stain removers are designed to eliminate these unsightly blemishes. (A severely stained pool may require professional acid washing to fully restore its beauty.) Meanwhile, sequestering agents and chelating formulas can be used to keep metals and organic material, respectively, from coming out of solution so that they can't settle and stain the pool or spa surface.

Solving Common Water Problems

WATER PROBLEM	DESCRIPTION
Algae	The most common type of alga is floating green. Other types include yellow/mustard and black (which is really a shade of dark blue). Algae can easily take root in pool walls and bloom quickly, sometimes within hours.
Cloudy water	Many things can cause cloudy water, including unbalanced water and poor filtration. Assuming the problem is water related and not the fault of equipment, the problem could be caused by algae, high levels of total dissolved solids (TDS), body oils, low sanitizer levels, or high pH or calcium hardness levels.
Stains	Stains can be caused by organic debris that gets into the water or by metals that come out of solution when the water isn't kept in balance. Copper can cause greenish blue, blue, or black stains. Iron stains are red or brown. Manganese stains are tan or purple. A gray stain, however, can mean a litany of things — from oxidized metal or scale deposits to moisture trapped in the plaster or even a trowel burn.
Scale	Scale occurs when minerals, especially calcium, come out of solution. The result is white, gray, or even brown deposits that mar the pool and spa surface and can damage equipment. Scale most often occurs when pH, total alkalinity, or calcium hardness levels are high.

COMMON WATER PROBLEMS AND SOLUTIONS

Most pool and spa water problems are easy to solve if you know what you're dealing with and the appropriate remedy for the situation. The following chart lists some of the more common water problems you may encounter, as well as advice for solving the problem and preventing it from happening again. If you can't find the solution to your water troubles here, don't hesitate to contact a professional pool and spa service technician, who should be able to help with even the most uncommon water-quality concerns.

SOLUTION	PREVENTION
An algaecide is the main artillery. Just make sure you're using an algaecide designed to combat your type of alga. Copper and silver are the most common active ingredients in algaecides, though there are some nonmetallic formulas that remove algae nutrients from the water, thereby starving the organisms. Of course, chlorine also kills algae. You might consider first brushing the algae from the pool wall to expose all of the cells to the algaecide. Green or yellow algae can be brushed away using a nylon or polyester brush, whereas black algae may require a wire brush.	Apply an algaecide regularly as recommended on the product label. Note that some products are designed to kill algae, others to prevent algae, and still others to do both. Make sure you're using the right product for the job at hand.
Shocking the water usually clears up any cloudiness, especially if the culprit is algae. If shocking doesn't work, use a clarifier to help the filtration system do its job.	Use a clarifier regularly, following the instructions on the product label. Make sure the clarifier you select is compatible with the sanitization system you're using.
Balance the water before treating the stain, or else it might occur again. Use a stain remover, available from your pool and spa supply store, that's designed to treat the type of stain you have. If your pool is plaster and is severely stained, you might need to consider draining the pool and having the surface acid-washed by a professional.	Keep the water balanced at all times. Use a stain preventive or metal remover when starting up your pool or spa and whenever fresh water is added.
Make sure the water is properly balanced. Then use a scale-removing product and thoroughly brush the walls to suspend the scale so the filter can trap it. You may need a special tile cleaner to remove scale deposits from the waterline area, where they're most noticeable.	Keep the water balanced at all times.

(chart continues)

Solving Common Water Problems

WATER PROBLEM	DESCRIPTION
Corrosive water	Corrosive water is acidic. It can damage pool and spa equipment and etch pool surfaces.
Alkaline water	Alkaline water is the opposite of corrosive water and usually results in the formation of scale. When the pH or alkalinity levels are too high, sanitizers don't work as effectively and cloudy water can result.
Eye and skin irritation	Improper pH levels are usually the cause of red, burning eyes, itchy skin, and rashes. An insufficient level of sanitizer, which allows the buildup of chloramines, can also be to blame.
Odor	Spa and pool owners often complain that their water has an unpleasant chlorine odor. It's a common misconception, however, that this odor is caused by having too much chlorine in the water. On the contrary, a strong chlorine odor means the water is producing chloramines. The presence of chloramines indicates an insufficient level of sanitizer; there's not enough sanitizer in the water to oxidize or burn away the chloramines.
Discolored water	Algae and metals are the most common causes of discolored water. Manganese, for example, can give the water a brown, black, or lavender hue. Copper can give the water a greenish tint. Iron can cause a brownish cast.
Foam	When the level of total dissolved solids is high and alkalinity is out of whack, pool and spa water tends to foam when agitated. Some algaecides also cause foaming. This is usually more of a problem in spas than in pools.
Scum	Scum is caused by a combination of contaminants, among them body oils, soaps, cosmetics, and lotions. Scum lines around your pool and spa are rarely harmful, but they can be gross.

SOLUTION	PREVENTION
Use soda ash (sometimes sold under a name like pH Up) or sodium bicarbonate to raise pH and total alkalinity.	Keep the water balanced at all times, paying special attention to pH and alkalinity.
Lower pH and total alkalinity by using a pH-reducing product. These include sodium bisulfate, sulfuric acid, hydrochloric acid, and muriatic acid. Consult your pool and spa supply dealer to find out which product is best for your particular situation. Sometimes the best way to lower pH is to replace some of the water with fresh water (assuming the source water isn't alkaline).	Keep the water balanced at all times, paying special attention to pH and alkalinity. If pH regularly drifts upward, routinely replace some of the water with fresh water to counter the introduction of bather waste, such as sweat, body oils, and sunscreen.
Test the water to find out whether any water-balance factors are out of their ideal range. Then shock the pool water to get rid of chloramines. (After shocking, keep swimmers out of the water until the chlorine residual drops below 10 ppm.)	Keep the water balanced at all times. Shock the water routinely to eliminate unwanted chloramines.
Test the water to find out whether any water-balance factors are out of their ideal range. Then shock the pool water to get rid of chloramines. (After shocking, keep swimmers out of the water until the chlorine residual drops below 10 ppm.)	Keep the water balanced at all times. Shock the water routinely to eliminate unwanted chloramines.
If the problem is algae, follow the guidelines for algae above. If a metal is the culprit, use a sequestering agent to keep the metal in solution. Also use a flocculant to cluster the metal particles so they're large enough to filter out.	Keep the water balanced at all times. If your source water has a high mineral content, use a metal remover (available from your pool and spa supply dealer) whenever you add fresh water to the pool or spa.
Use a small amount of defoamer and allow it to circulate for several minutes before adding more as needed. For a long-term solution, balance, shock, and/or replace some of the water with fresh water.	Keep the water balanced at all times. Ask bathers to shower before entering the pool or spa to minimize contaminants in the water. Change spa water completely every two to three months, depending on the bather load.
Use an over-the-counter tub and tile cleaner to scrub away the scum. Use as little as possible to minimize the amount of cleaner entering the water.	Have swimmers and bathers shower before entering the pool or spa. Use a scum-absorbing product (available from pool and spa supply stores) that traps scum before it has a chance to cling to the pool or spa walls.

6

Cleaning a Pool

onsumer surveys tell us that one of the biggest deterrents to buying a swimming pool is maintenance. While everyone would rather relax poolside than jockey a vacuum pole, routine maintenance is a reality for every pool owner. Fortunately, the task is much easier if you invest in an automatic pool cleaner (APC). The up-front cost of this unit will save you countless hours over the lifetime of your pool.

Many new pool owners underestimate the time involved in manually vacuuming their pool and later convert to automatic pool cleaners. This conversion process is much easier if your pool is plumbed during the construction process to handle one of the automatic cleaners. Many pool builders assume that their customers will eventually opt to purchase an automatic pool cleaner after a couple of years of manual cleaning and routinely make their pools APC compatible during construction.

The best way to simplify your pool-cleaning regimen — whether you're using manual or automatic pool cleaning equipment — is to maintain the pool properly between cleanings. See appendix A for details.

CLEANING TOOLS

Before you begin cleaning the pool, assemble all the tools you'll need. Otherwise you'll end up running back and forth to the pool storage area as you progress through the cleaning process. Here's a list of essential equipment.

Telescoping Poles

Telescoping poles, sometimes called telepoles, are a must-have item for pool owners. They're made from aluminum or fiberglass and consist of an outer cylinder that slides over an inner cylinder, so that the pole can be extended to twice the length it is when retracted. An 8-foot (2.4 m) pool that extends to 16 feet (4.9 m) should suit most of your pool-cleaning needs. The two cylinders usually lock together with a cam lock or a compression nut ring.

The tip of the pole may be fitted with a magnet to help you pick up metal objects, such as hairpins, that fall to the pool floor. Various attachments — such as vacuum heads and brushes — can be installed on the end of a tele-scoping pole. Some tools insert into the pole, while others slide over the pole. The attachments have locking devices that secure them to the pole.

Rakes

A pool rake is a small, sturdy net used in conjunction with a telescoping pole to remove leaves and other floating debris from the pool. The net can be made from stainless-steel mesh or plastic netting, and its frame is usually aluminum or plastic. There are many different kinds of pool rakes available; invest in a good-quality rake that will withstand being scraped against rough surfaces and lifting heavy loads of wet debris.

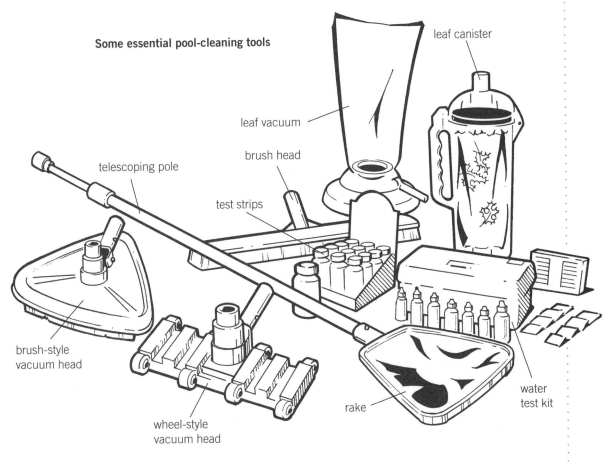

Some essential pool-cleaning tools

leaf canister

leaf vacuum

brush head

telescoping pole

test strips

brush-style vacuum head

wheel-style vacuum head

rake

water test kit

Brushes

Nylon-bristled wall and floor brushes are used in conjunction with a telescoping pole to remove dirt, stains, and other foreign matter from the pool's interior surfaces. Most are about 18 inches (46 cm) wide; some are curved for easier access to corners and other tight crevices.

To remove tough stains and algae, you'll need a brush with stainless-steel bristles.

Tile Brushes

Tile brushes usually have abrasive foam pads and snap into a telescoping pole so you can scrub the tile without getting down on your hands and knees. Use these brushes with cleansing formulas designed for pool tile, available from your pool and spa supply store. Other types of cleansers or soaps foam excessively and can wreak havoc on your pool's circulation system.

Pumice Stones

Pumice is handy for removing scale, stains, and menacing deposits from tile and plasters without excessive scratching. It's sold in block form or as a bladed stone that attaches to a telescoping pool.

Water Test Kits and Chemicals

After you've cleaned the pool, you'll need to test and balance the water.

Vacuum

You'll need a vacuum to suck up debris from the bottom of the pool. Pool vacuums come in two different categories: manual and automatic.

MANUAL VACUUMS

Two types of manual vacuum heads are used to clean debris from pools: Suction-style vacuums suck debris into the pool's filtration system; leaf vacuums use water pressure supplied by a garden hose to force debris into a mesh bag. Both types attach to a telescoping pole.

Like household vacuum cleaners, many pool vacuums have adjustable heads that can be set to maintain a specific distance from the pool surface, enabling you to achieve maximal effectiveness for your pool surface. Some vacuum heads glide on bristles, while others incorporate wheels. Make sure you're using a type designed for your pool surface; wheels, for example, can damage a vinyl-lined pool.

Suction-Style Vacuums

The suction-style vacuum features a hose attached at one end to the vacuum head and at the other end to a special port below the pool's skimmer. When you turn on the filter pump, water is pulled from the vacuum head to the skimmer, where debris is filtered out. The vacuum hose is available in many lengths; make sure you have one that is long enough to reach every corner of your pool. Some hoses have swivel cuffs, which help prevent the hose from coiling or kinking while you work.

Before you start vacuuming, make sure all the suction power of your pool's circulation system is concentrated at the port in the wall where you attach the vacuum hose. You may need to consult with a pool service technician the first time you do this to make sure you're closing off main drains and multiple skimmers correctly to create the suction required. Also make sure the hose is filled with water before attaching it to the suction port. If too much air is allowed into the circulation system, the pump could lose its prime and stop operating.

Attach the vacuum head to a telescoping pole and work your way slowly around the pool. Don't move too fast, or else you'll merely stir up debris instead of vacuuming it up. If the suction becomes weak, clean the pump strainer basket and filter. When you're finished, remove the end of the hose from the suction port and lift the vacuum head from the water, allowing the water in the hose to drain back into the pool.

Leaf Vacuums

A leaf vacuum, which has its own filter, is designed to pick up large amounts of debris, but it won't pick up the finer particles that a suction-style vacuum will collect. Despite its limitations, a leaf vacuum can be handy, particularly if you have lots of debris (such as leaves) to clean out and you don't want to have to stop every few minutes to clean out your skimmer basket. After you've used a leaf vacuum to clean out the big stuff, you can follow up with a suction-style vacuum to finish the job.

To operate a leaf-style vacuum, you'll attach a garden hose to a water supply (presumably your outdoor spigot) at one end and to the vacuum head at the other end, and then attach the vacuum head to a telescoping pole. Place the vacuum in the pool and turn on the water. Move the vacuum head around the pool to pick up

If there are lots of leaves in your pool, you may want to attach a leaf canister to the hose of your suction-style vacuum. A leaf canister traps leaves while allowing water to pass through to the filter, so you don't have to empty the pump strainer basket as often.

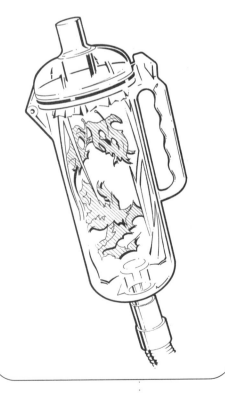

leaves and large debris, stopping to empty the leaf bag as needed. When you're finished, remove the vacuum carefully from the water to avoid spilling debris back into the pool. (You may wish to leave the water on until the vacuum is removed from the pool.) Then clean out the leaf bag.

If your garden hose has weak water pressure, a leaf vacuum may not perform well.

AUTOMATIC POOL CLEANERS

Using an automatic pool cleaner (APC) can save you about three hours a week in routine chores. Plus, APCs help pool water stay warmer by circulating cooler water to the surface, where it is warmed by the sun; conserve water by lowering the temperature of the surface water, thereby making it less vulnerable to evaporation; and save chemicals by helping distribute them evenly throughout the pool.

That said, it should come as no surprise that APCs have moved to the front and center of the war against sunken debris and tile scum. In fact, many pool owners now consider an APC a necessity rather than a luxury.

Before you run out and buy an APC, you should know that there are several types, and each works best on particular pool surfaces. For example, you wouldn't want to use a cleaner designed to scrub plaster surfaces if you have a vinyl-lined pool, or you may end up having to replace the liner sooner than you thought. Also, some units are sized for smaller aboveground pools; if you used one of these on your massive in-ground pool, you'd be disappointed with the results.

The basic types of pool cleaners include suction, pressure, electric, and in-floor. Here's a brief description of each.

Suction

Suction cleaners are the least expensive type of pool cleaner. Simple to operate, they attach to the suction side of the pool's plumbing system — the side that brings water out of the pool to be filtered. A hose connects the cleaner to one of the pool's suction ports. This is usually the skimmer, though more and more new pools are being constructed with a separate vacuum port for the cleaner's hose.

When the filter pump is running, suction is created on the underside of the cleaner. The cleaner then moves randomly around the pool, sucking up debris. Large debris is caught in the pump's strainer basket; small debris passes through to the pool's filter, where it is trapped. Some tweaking of the device and the pool circulation system is necessary to achieve optimal coverage of the pool floor and walls.

The main problem with suction cleaners occurs in pools that have only one skimmer. In this situation, skimmer action must be suspended while the cleaner is operating, which means floating debris won't be removed while the vacuum is connected. Also, unless you have an in-line strainer basket on the hose, the filter pump basket can fill up quickly, depending on how much debris has fallen into the pool.

If a suction cleaner is not moving as it should, check to ensure that the main drain and all suction lines except the one the cleaner is attached to are closed. Also remove any debris from the pump basket, and check the opening to the cleaner and remove any obstructions, such as leaves. Obstructions can also be found where the hose attaches to the suction line.

The cleaner may move slowly if air is getting into the hose, so check the hose for cracks, splits, or holes. Air can also get into the system via a loose or cracked pump basket lid. Air bubbles entering the pool at the return line are a sure sign that air is getting into the vacuum system.

Suction cleaners require a minimum flow rate to work effectively. If nothing appears to be wrong with the cleaner, consult your pool professional to make sure your pool's circulation system is adequately sized for the cleaner you're trying to use.

Suction-side cleaners draw debris to the filtration system, where it's trapped by the pump strainer basket and filter.

Pressure-side cleaners use water pressure from a garden hose or pool return line to force dirt and debris into a filter bag.

Pressure

Pressure cleaners attach to the pressure side of your pool's circulation system — that is, the side that returns water to the pool after it's been filtered. These units attach to an exiting return inlet or a dedicated port. The pressure from the water powers the cleaner. As water flows toward the unit, it is split into three directions: the sweeper tail, the thrust jet, and the venturi.

The sweeper tail helps stir up fine debris from the floor and walls so that it can be caught in the pool's main filter. The thrust jet is a series of ports and gears that send the cleaner around the pool in a random pattern. The venturi is a port to which a filter bag is attached. As water flows through the venturi, larger debris is trapped in the filter bag. The filter bag must be emptied when full.

Some pressure cleaners require a booster pump in order to ensure enough pressure power is created by the circulation system. In such cases, it's best to have the booster pump installed during the pool construction process so that the dedicated line from the booster pump can be installed under the deck and through the pool wall.

Your pool dealer should be able to help you test the pressure at the inlet port to determine whether your pool's circulation system provides enough pressure to power one of these cleaners without the need for a booster pump. One advantage of systems that do require booster pumps, however, is that the booster pump can be set on a timer, so if the cleaner is left in the pool, the cleaning system is truly automatic.

One of the advantages of pressure cleaners in general is that they help distribute clean, filtered, and chemically treated water around the pool. Also, because they have their own filter bag to capture debris, they don't cause excessive wear on the pool's main filtration system. And a pressure cleaner will operate even when its filter bag is full; water still flows through the cleaner and stirs up debris, and the filter bag just won't collect any more until it is emptied. If the debris were being caught in the pump filter basket — as it is with suction-style cleaners — the pool's pump would have to work harder to keep circulating water.

Electric

Sometimes referred to as robot cleaners, electric cleaners are low-voltage devices that hook up to a standard GFCI-protected outlet. A transformer converts the electrical power to a voltage that is strong enough to power the unit but low enough not to create a danger of electrocution. These cleaners come with long — about 50 feet (15 m) — electrical cords to ensure that the cleaner can reach the entire pool.

Electric cleaners typically have two motors. The pump motor sucks up water and debris into the cleaner's filter; the drive motor moves the unit around the pool. The onboard filter is easy to clean. To improve performance, some of these units are controlled via a computerized system, which can be programmed to remember the shape and size of the pool. Some units even have remote control capabilities, so you can drive the cleaner around the pool from your poolside lounge chair.

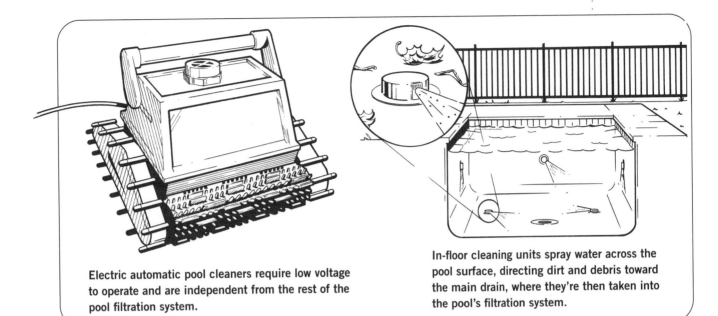

Electric automatic pool cleaners require low voltage to operate and are independent from the rest of the pool filtration system.

In-floor cleaning units spray water across the pool surface, directing dirt and debris toward the main drain, where they're then taken into the pool's filtration system.

The biggest advantage of electric cleaners is that they're independent from the rest of the pool circulation system, so they don't create any problems for the regular filtration process. However, they can cost a lot more than either suction or pressure cleaners.

Never pull an electric cleaner out of the water by its cord, or you risk causing a short in the wiring. Instead, always reach into the pool and lift the cleaner out by its handle.

If a unit moves along the pool floor but doesn't suck up any debris, the pump motor may be shorted out. If water is gushing from the cleaner but it won't move, the problem may lie with the drive motor. In either case — and with all malfunctions in an electrical cleaner — it's best to have repairs made by one of the manufacturer's authorized service centers.

In-Floor

An in-floor cleaning system can be installed only during the construction of a pool. In-floor systems are more expensive than the other types of APCs but also offer the greatest ease of use. Essentially, an in-floor cleaning system consists of multiple jets installed in the pool floor, steps, and other underwater surfaces where debris is likely to rest. When the system is activated, these rotating jets project high-pressure streams of water that "sweep" sediment and debris along the floor and walls toward the pool's main drain, where they can be removed by the pool's filtration system.

Because of how they operate, in-floor cleaning systems are custom designed for each pool to ensure top performance.

Troubleshooting Automatic Pool Cleaners

When you purchase an automatic pool cleaner, keep the owner's manual handy. Here you'll find instructions for proper care and operation of your pool cleaner, as well as troubleshooting tips should something go wrong. Also, many manufacturers offer troubleshooting advice on their Web sites.

To alleviate wear and tear and to prevent breakdowns, check your cleaner periodically to make sure it's working properly and fix any small glitches before they develop into major problems. Always replace worn parts, or else you risk having to replace more expensive components down the road.

Though it's impossible to predict everything that might go wrong with an automatic pool cleaner, some general advice for improving the performance of your cleaner may be of assistance.

- Make sure the cleaner you purchase is designed for the type and size of pool you own.
- Make sure the hose (or electric cord) is long enough to reach every section of the pool easily.
- If the cleaner misses spots or gets stuck, make sure the strong current from the return jets isn't forcing the cleaner into a pattern or preventing it from moving. To remedy this situation, adjust the return fittings or replace them with adjustable eyeball diverters that you can angle in different directions. In most cases, it helps to angle the fittings downward.
- Make sure proper vacuum pressure is maintained at all time. Vacuum pressure is affected by clogs in filters, skimmer baskets, and pump baskets. Air leaks in the hose, pump basket lid, or other points along the circulation system can also cause a drop in pressure.
- To keep hoses from twisting, don't coil them up for storage. If possible, allow the hose sections to lie flat. Hoses perform best when they're straight. If you do have a coiled hose, stretch it out in the sun for an entire day to relax the coils.
- Cleaners will have trouble climbing walls coated with slippery algae. Maintain the proper water chemistry at all times and brush walls thoroughly. Many cleaners also have trouble climbing walls if the angle where the wall and floor meet is sharp and not sloped.
- If the cleaner moves too quickly or too slowly, check the pressure at the inlet or outlet (depending on whether you're using a suction or pressure cleaner) to make sure it's in the range recommended by the manufacturer.
- Don't use an automatic pool cleaner on a newly plastered pool until it's had at least three weeks to cure or the cleaner will mar the surface.

STEP-BY-STEP POOL CLEANING

Cleaning a pool is a simple matter of following a few basic steps.

1. Clean the deck area so that debris doesn't blow or get tracked into your newly cleaned pool and spa.

2. Use a leaf rake to remove floating debris, emptying the rake into a garbage bag as needed. Don't dispose of the debris you collect in your garden, because it might blow back into your pool when it dries out. Also, the small amount of chemicals in the wet debris could be harmful to your plants. You may need to rake daily if your pool tends to collect a lot of blowing leaves and debris.

3. Use tile brushes and an appropriate tile cleaner to clean the tile surfaces of your pool. Be sure to scrub both above and below the waterline. If necessary, use a pumice stone to remove stains. (It's important to clean the tile before the rest of the pool because debris scrubbed from the tiles, as well as particles from a pumice stone, will settle to the bottom as you clean. You can vacuum up these particles later.) Some automatic pool cleaners claim to brush the waterline for you, but they won't do a perfect job or reach tight corners. Needless to say, a little elbow grease is always needed.

4. Bring the water level up to where it should be. You may need to add water weekly to compensate for evaporation and "splash out." If you have an automatic water leveler attached to your pool, it should do the job for you.

5. Empty and clean the skimmer basket and the pump strainer basket. Then check the filter's pressure. If the filter pressure is high, you may need to clean it before vacuuming. Also take this time to clean the area around the equipment pad. Observe the equipment to make sure everything is operating as it should. Look for leaks.

6. Brush the pool walls. Brushing removes algae from the walls and helps expose them to the sanitizing chemicals in the water. Start at the shallow end and work toward the deep end, brushing toward the main drain so that debris is sucked into the filtration system. Some automatic cleaners climb walls and brush them for you, but again, they never do a perfect job or reach tight spaces. If you have one of these cleaners, you should manually brush the spots your cleaner usually misses.

7. If debris is visible on the bottom of the pool, vacuum the pool using either a manual or an automatic pool cleaner.

If you use a suction-style cleaner, clean the pump strainer basket and filter again after vacuuming.

8. Perform routine water tests, as described in chapter 4. Balance the water and add sanitizing chemicals as needed.

7

Pool and Spa Filtration

 pool or spa filter acts like a human kidney, cleaning water that circulates through it. Without a filter, the water would be murky, cloudy, difficult to sanitize, and generally unsuitable for swimming or bathing. The earliest swimming pools didn't have the luxury of filtration, and the only way to clarify the water was to replace all or part of it with fresh water. Today, refilling the pool or spa every time you wanted to use it would be not only inconvenient but also costly and un-ecological. By filtering pool and spa water, we're able to conserve water, reduce chemical use, and maintain a healthy swimming environment.

A properly filtered and chemically treated spa may still need to be drained and refilled once every two to three months. A well-maintained pool, on the other hand, will need fresh water added only to replace water lost to evaporation, filter cleaning, and splashing from normal use.

There are three types of filters commonly available to pool and spa owners: sand, diatomaceous earth (DE), and cartridge. Most portable spas and above-ground pools use cartridge filters; all three types of filters are popular for in-ground pools. Each type of filter has its advantages and disadvantages; you should be familiar with all of them to make sure you're using the best filter for your particular pool and spa setup. In general, DE costs the most but filters out the smallest particles. Sand costs the least but does the least effective job. Cartridges fall somewhere in the middle.

The effectiveness of a filter is gauged by the smallness of particles it can screen out. For this purpose, particles are measured in microns. A *micron* is a unit of linear measurement equivalent to one millionth of a meter. Though manufacturers will argue about the effectiveness of their filter medium over others, as a general guide you can assume that sand will filter particles down to 20 to 40 microns, cartridges will filter down to 10 to 20 microns, and DE will filter down to 2 to 5 microns. As a means of comparison, a grain of salt is 90 to 110 microns wide, and particles under 35 microns can't be seen with the naked eye. Even so, particles smaller than 1 micron can make water appear cloudy if there are enough of them.

That said, here's a detailed look at each filter type.

SAND FILTERS

Granules of sand are irregularly shaped and make an efficient filtering medium, as evidenced by the many freshwater creeks that are naturally filtered by sand. Sand filters contain a deep layer of sand that traps dirt and debris as water flows through it. The trapped particles fill the spaces between granules of sand and actually help the filter collect even smaller particles.

Over time, the accumulation of trapped particles will restrict water flow, the pressure inside the filter will increase, and it will be time to backwash, or clean, the filter. Backwashing simply calls for reversing the flow of water through the filter tank to loosen the trapped dirt so that it can be washed away.

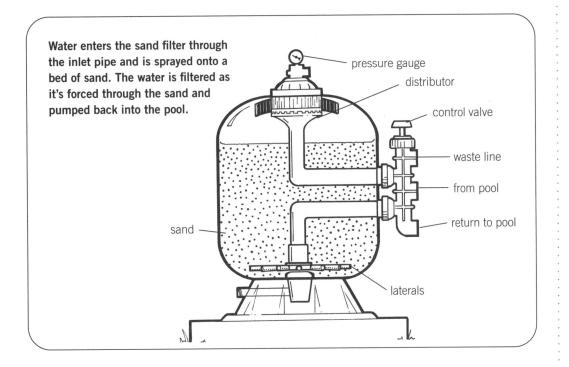

Water enters the sand filter through the inlet pipe and is sprayed onto a bed of sand. The water is filtered as it's forced through the sand and pumped back into the pool.

pressure gauge
distributor
control valve
waste line
from pool
return to pool
sand
laterals

The amount of dirt a filter can hold depends on how large the sand bed within the filter is. You want to put the maximum amount of sand in the filter that's recommended, but make sure to leave a space between the top of the sand bed and the lowest opening in the distributor (where the water enters the filter). This space, called the *freeboard*, should be at least half the depth of the sand bed. Because every sand filter is unique, check the manufacturer's recommendations for proper operation.

Sand filters require a particular type of sand. Check your owner's manual for the correct sand specifications. If the grain of sand is too large or too small, the filter will not run efficiently and may even become damaged.

Backwashing

Many sand filters are fitted with two pressure gauges: the inlet gauge and the outlet gauge. When the sand is clean, the difference between the two gauges is usually about 3 psi (pounds per square inch). As the sand becomes dirty, however, the pressure on the inlet gauge will increase while the pressure on the outlet gauge will decrease. Most manufacturers recommend that you backwash the filter when the difference between the two gauges is 18 to 20 psi.

If your filter has just one gauge (it will be on the inlet), you'll need to take note of the starting pressure the first time the system is turned on with clean sand in it. The filter may have the projected starting pressure stamped on it, but don't rely on this estimate to determine when it's time to backwash. Instead, record the *actual* starting pressure. When the inlet gauge shows an increase of 8 to 10 psi over the starting pressure, it's time to backwash the filter.

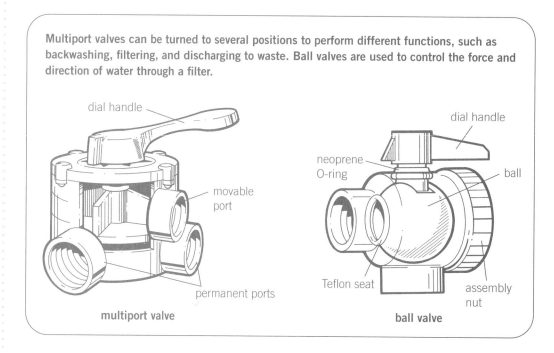

Multiport valves can be turned to several positions to perform different functions, such as backwashing, filtering, and discharging to waste. Ball valves are used to control the force and direction of water through a filter.

dial handle

movable port

permanent ports

multiport valve

dial handle

neoprene O-ring

ball

Teflon seat

assembly nut

ball valve

To backwash a sand filter, turn the control valve to "backwash" and divert the outlet water to the "waste" line. This will reverse the flow of water through the sand bed, thereby loosening dirt particles so the water can carry them away to the waste line. The process usually takes 2 to 4 minutes. Some waste lines are plumbed with a sight glass so that you can observe the water as it's flowing through to make sure the water is clean before you end the backwashing cycle.

When the backwashing is complete, turn off the pump so that the redistributed sand can settle in the tank. If you have a filter-to-waste option on your filter, use it now. This allows you to divert the first 20 seconds or so of filtered water to the waste line to make sure that no settled dirt that was missed during the backwash cycle is able to enter the pool. Once this is done, you can switch to regular filtration. If you don't have the filter-to-waste option, you might see a puff of dirt and debris enter the pool when you first start up the pool following a backwash cycle.

Improving Performance

Flocculants are often used to improve the performance of sand filters. As an alternative, diatomaceous earth can be used so long as long your municipality doesn't prohibit the discharge of DE during the backwash process. If DE is acceptable, pour 0.5 cup (0.12 L) of DE for every 3 square feet (0.28 m²) of filter area into the filter after the unit has been filled with sand.

Eventually the rough sand in your filter will become smooth and you'll need to replace it. Sand is usually good for a few years, but you'll know it's time for a change when the filter's effectiveness becomes greatly diminished. To change the sand, simply turn off the power, open the filter, and scoop out the old sand by hand. Then fill the bottom third of the tank with water to cushion the impact of new sand on the laterals (the pipes that carry filtered water out of the filter). Fill the tank about two-thirds full with sand. Reassemble the filter and backwash for several seconds to remove any impurities from the sand, then filter as normal.

GIVE IT TIME

Don't backwash any more than is recommended by the manufacturer of your filter. If you backwash too frequently, you're not giving the filter the opportunity to do an efficient job. Remember, you need some dirt in the filter in order for the filter to trap the smaller particles.

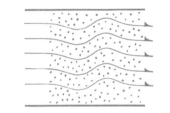

When the sand in the filter is clean, water passes through easily.

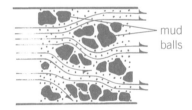

mud balls

When pool water is unbalanced and the filter isn't cleaned properly, mud balls can form and impede the filtering process.

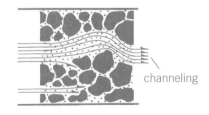

channeling

As the situation worsens, the water forces channels through the sand, allowing unfiltered water to pass back into the pool.

DIATOMACEOUS EARTH FILTERS

Diatomaceous earth filters produce sparkling clear pool and spa water because they're capable of filtering out even the smallest particles. This level of quality explains why DE filters cost the most to operate.

As the name implies, DE filters use diatomaceous earth as a filtering medium. DE is a fine, chalky powder made from the fossilized remains of microscopic sea organisms (diatoms). DE is mined from large deposits found where ancient inland seas have dried up. These deposits take the form of soft rock, which is pulverized to produce a fine, talcum-like powder. Though DE may feel soft, it actually has an incredibly large number of microscopic jagged edges that help it trap extremely small particles when used as a filtering medium. The dusty nature of DE, however, means that users must take special care not to inhale the dry material. In fact, DE is a known carcinogen, and many municipalities don't allow residents to discharge used DE into the municipal wastewater system. (To check out the regulations in your area, contact your local health department.) If used properly, however, DE is as safe as it is effective.

The inside of a DE filter is very different from that of a sand filter. Inside the filter tank are grids covered with a polypropylene cloth. A typical filter has eight grids that total 24 to 72 square feet (2.2 to 6.7 m²). There are two basic types of grids: vertical and spin.

- ~ **Vertical grid filters** have grids assembled vertically on a manifold. A holding wheel secures the grids to the manifold and a retaining rod screws into the base of the tank to secure the assembly. Water enters the tank at the bottom. It flows up and around the outside of the grids and then down the stem of each grid, into the hollow manifold, and out of the filter.
- ~ **Spin grid filters** are now obsolete but may still be found in older pools. The grids are shaped like wheels and line up horizontally like a box of doughnuts. They operate in a manner similar to that of vertical grid filters, but they're not as effective. To clean the grids, the user must turn a crank to spin them.

Once the filter is assembled and the pool's circulation system is turned on, you'll pour a thin slurry of DE and water through the skimmer basket. The slurry ends up in the filter, where the DE coats the grid cloth, which is woven tight enough to keep the DE from passing through. This layer of DE — ideally $\frac{1}{16}$ to $\frac{1}{8}$ inch thick — does the actual filtering, not the grid cloth.

To avoid damage to the grids — which are costly to repair — make sure you add the right amount of DE for the type and size of filter you have. The owner's manual for the filter should specify the proper amount of DE to use and how to prepare the slurry mixture.

Backwashing

As the DE traps dirt and debris from the pool water passing through it, the pressure inside the filter increases. When the pressure gauge (located on the top or side of the filter) reaches the level specified by the manufacturer, it's time to backwash the filter, following the instructions in the owner's manual.

During the backwash cycle, water flows up through the filter and dislodges the cake of DE and dirt from the filter grids. The DE and debris are flushed into the waste line. After the backwash cycle is through, a fresh slurry of DE and water is added through the skimmer basket to recoat the filter grids. It's important that all DE be backwashed to waste during the cleaning process. If DE is allowed to remain in

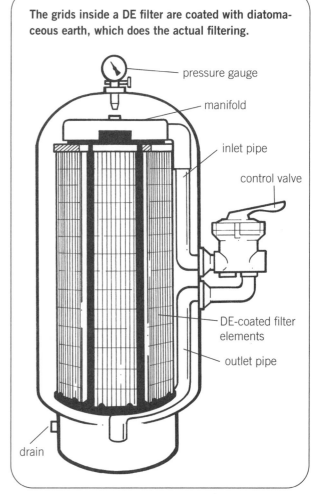

The grids inside a DE filter are coated with diatomaceous earth, which does the actual filtering.

pressure gauge

manifold

inlet pipe

control valve

DE-coated filter elements

outlet pipe

drain

the filter, adding new DE will result in too much DE, which could cause *bridging,* a situation wherein DE and dirt close the necessary gap between the filter grids, reducing the flow rate as well as the square footage of the filter area.

DE Disposal

If your municipality doesn't permit DE to be flushed into the waste-water system, you'll need to fit your filter with a separation tank. This tank is smaller than the filter and is equipped with a mesh bag or other screening device that filters the DE out of the wastewater. The DE can then be easily removed and disposed of properly, either with the regular trash or through a hazardous waste disposal site.

Regenerative DE Filters

Many DE filters available today are regenerative. This means you can redistribute the DE when the filter becomes clogged so that clean particles of DE are exposed, thereby extending the life of the DE.

How do you redistribute the DE in the filter? Most regenerative DE filters have a handle on the top. Every few days, you should turn off the pump and move the handle up and down according to the manufacturer's directions. Other filter designs call for rotating the grid assembly. Whatever the design, the objective is the same: to dislodge the DE cake and allow the DE to redistribute itself when the pump is turned back on.

If after regenerating the DE the filter pressure doesn't drop back down to the starting pressure, it may be time to replace the DE.

Washing the DE Grids

Sometimes it may be necessary to remove and wash the grid elements to clean away body oils, embedded dirt, and calcium deposits. You'll know it's time to clean the grids when the filtration cycle is shorter than usual or the pressure in the filter doesn't return to normal after backwashing. One common method is to acid-wash each of the grids in a 25 percent solution of muriatic acid (one part acid to four parts water). After soaking the grids in the solution, rinse them thoroughly with fresh water. Overexposing the grids to acid can damage the elements, so make sure you rinse them immediately after cleaning.

Before reassembling a DE filter, inspect the inside and remove any debris. Carefully look at each grid for damage. If there's a small hole in the filter element, you might be able to repair it with fingernail polish or silicone sealer. If you don't, DE will wash through the grid and enter the pool. If the hole is too big to repair this way, you'll need to replace the entire grid.

CARTRIDGE FILTERS

Because of their ease of maintenance, cartridge filters are growing in popularity for all types of pools and spas. Unlike sand and DE filters, cartridge filters don't need to be backwashed. The cartridge filtering medium — a cylinder of pleated, polyester fabric — can be removed and hosed off when it becomes clogged. Not only does this conserve water, it also saves on pool chemicals because you're not backwashing treated pool water down the drain.

The cartridge filter is housed inside a tank or canister. Water is drawn into the tank, passes through the filter, which traps dirt and debris, and then travels back into the pool.

The effectiveness of a cartridge filter depends greatly on the quality and size of the cartridge. Cartridges are differentiated by the weight of the polyester fabric, the overall square footage of the fabric, the depth of the pleats in the fabric, and the type of end cap construction.

Most manufacturers use a 4-ounce fabric, although a 6-ounce material is more effective for filtering small particles. However, the lighter-weight material costs less, and a cartridge can hold more square footage of 4-ounce material than of 6-ounce material, increasing its effectiveness. You might find some cartridges using 3-ounce material, but their effectiveness will be greatly reduced, even though they contain more square footage of material. A 3-ounce filter might suffice for a spa application, but it won't be adequate for a swimming pool.

Though greater square footage of filtering medium can mean better filtration, it's not necessarily the case if the pleats of the fabric are crammed so tightly together that water has difficulty flowing through them. In essence, if you put too much fabric in a filter, you restrict the flow of water and hinder the filter's performance. To increase the filtering square footage without squeezing the fabric too tightly, some filter canisters are designed to hold two or three cartridges.

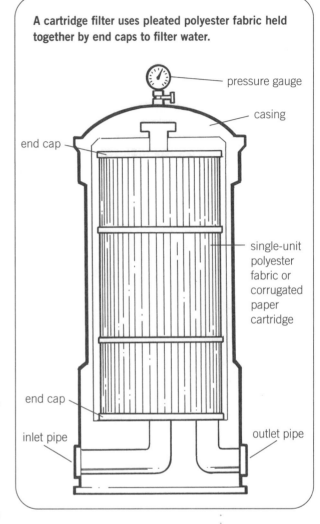

A cartridge filter uses pleated polyester fabric held together by end caps to filter water.

- pressure gauge
- casing
- end cap
- single-unit polyester fabric or corrugated paper cartridge
- end cap
- inlet pipe
- outlet pipe

Pleats that are too deep — more than 2.5 inches (6 cm) — also reduce the effectiveness of a cartridge filter. Water always seeks the path of least resistance. As a pleat in a cartridge becomes clogged with dirt, the water works its way up the pleat and into adjacent pleats. If the pleats are too deep, the water is trapped in them and the flow is restricted.

Cartridge end caps are designed to fit specific filter applications. Some need to pull double duty by supporting the pleated filter medium and creating a tight seal when placed in the canister. Be sure to check the cartridge's end cap design, not just the overall dimensions, when purchasing replacement cartridges.

Cleaning the Cartridge

As with other types of filters, a cartridge filter should be cleaned when the pressure gauge on top of the unit reads 8 to 10 psi above the filter's starting pressure. Unlike other filter types, however, cartridge filters don't require backwashing. The basic steps for cleaning a cartridge filter are as follows:

1. Remove the filter from the canister or filter tank according to the manufacturer's instructions.

2. Using a garden hose with a straight-flow nozzle, spray water through the fabric to remove dirt. Work from the top down, making sure to spray between the pleats where dirt and debris build up. Rinse the cartridge until all the dirt and debris appears to be gone.

3. Replace the cartridge in the canister or tank.

If the filter has been exposed to heavy bather loads or high levels of perspiration and body oils (which is especially common with spas), you may need to soak it in a cleaning solution overnight after hosing it down. You can purchase a filter-cleaning product from a pool and spa supply store, or you can use 1 cup (0.24 L) of trisodium phosphate or dishwasher detergent mixed with 5 gallons (18.9 L) of water. After soaking, rinse the cartridge thoroughly.

If the filter is coated with algae or calcium deposits, you may need to acid-wash it. Do not attempt to acid-wash a cartridge filter without first removing all oils and subsequent cleaning solution. Otherwise the acid will destroy the filter element. When you are ready to acid-wash, prepare a solution of 1 part muriatic acid mixed with 20 parts water. Soak the cartridge in the acid solution just until the solution stops bubbling. Then rinse the cartridge thoroughly and immediately place it back in the canister or tank.

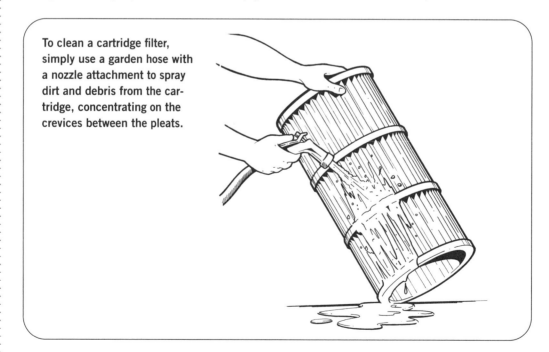

To clean a cartridge filter, simply use a garden hose with a nozzle attachment to spray dirt and debris from the cartridge, concentrating on the crevices between the pleats.

Replacing Cartridges

In terms of life expectancy, cartridges can be expected to last one to six years, depending on the quality of the cartridge and the care it's been given. Replace cartridges when they're no longer cleanable, when the webbing of the fabric appears shiny and closed, or when the fabric has begun to deteriorate or tear.

To extend the life of your cartridge filter, consider having your vacuum line run directly to waste rather than through the filter. Sometimes a heavy and sudden dirt load can clog and even damage the cartridge.

SIZING A FILTER CORRECTLY

No matter what kind of filter system you choose — sand, DE, or cartridge — the filter must be sized to the volume of water in your pool or spa. The basic rule is to size the pump and motor to the pool or spa capacity, then size the filter (its flow rate and capacity) to the pump.

For a pool, the recommended *turnover time* (the time it takes for the pump to circulate the entire body of water) is about eight hours. An eight-hour turnover time does not necessarily mean the filtration system must run eight hours daily to ensure clean water. In fact, if your pool water is correctly balanced and has the recommended levels of free or available sanitizer, you may find that you can reduce filtration cycles to six, four, and sometimes as little as two hours per day. But short filtration cycles must conform to individual pool conditions and requirements, which may vary from season to season. A professional pool equipment dealer or pool builder can help you figure out the right filter size and filtration cycle for your pool or spa.

In many cities and counties throughout the United States, filter rates on pools (especially commercial pools) are regulated. The faster water passes through the filter medium, the less effectively it's cleaned. Thus, to ensure effective filtration, the National Sanitation Foundation offers recommendations for maximum filter rates, which may or may not be adopted by local building codes.

Just remember, if the filter is too small, it won't keep the pool clean. If the filter is too large, it will cost more to buy but not necessarily more to operate. So don't opt for the minimum-size filter to fit your requirements. Such a filter may work fine under normal conditions, but any sudden influx of dirt and debris from heavy rain and wind could quickly overload it. You're better off

> ## USING THE PRESSURE-RELEASE VALVE
>
> All types of filters have a pressure-release valve. You must release this valve before turning on the pump. When a steady stream of water shoots out of the filter, close the valve. The pressure-release valve allows air inside the filter to escape as water begins rushing through the canister. If you don't open the pressure-release valve, the air pressure inside the filter builds. If the air pressure becomes too great, the filter can explode.

slightly oversizing the filter than using a filter that is too small for the pool. If you oversize the filter, make sure the pump is sized accordingly, because a pump that is too small for the filter may not backwash it adequately.

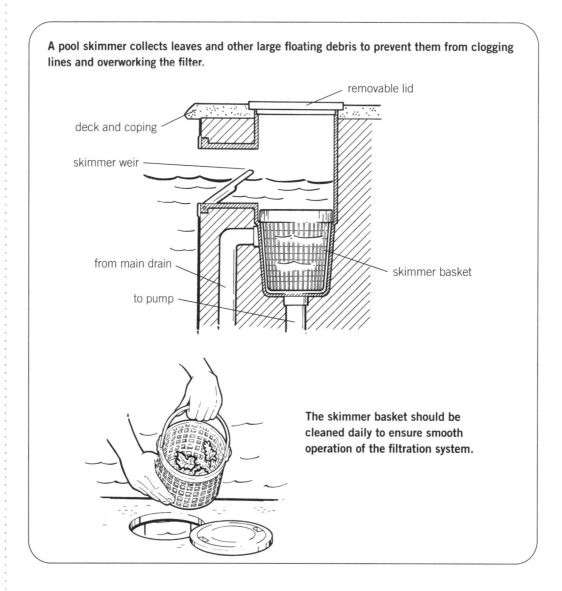

A pool skimmer collects leaves and other large floating debris to prevent them from clogging lines and overworking the filter.

removable lid

deck and coping

skimmer weir

from main drain

to pump

skimmer basket

The skimmer basket should be cleaned daily to ensure smooth operation of the filtration system.

TROUBLESHOOTING

When something goes wrong with your pool or spa filtration system, water quality can deteriorate quickly. Poor filtration also leads to increased chemical costs and a greater need for sanitizer. Following are some basic filter problems and possible solutions. For the most part, problems affect all filter types — sand, DE, and cartridge. As always, these guidelines are for general information only. Be sure to consult the owner's manual for your filter for specific recommendations and operating guidelines.

Troubleshooting the Filter

PROBLEM	POSSIBLE CAUSES	SOLUTION
Pressure-gauge needle won't move when the filtration system is turned on or off.	Pressure gauge is stuck.	Tap the face or casing of the gauge firmly to dislodge the stuck needle. If the gauge doesn't register water pressure, it won't be possible to monitor the filter's performance. Also, excessively high filter pressure can lead to filter damage and personal injury. Replace the filter gauge if it doesn't immediately begin working properly.
Flow rate is low.	Accumulated dirt is restricting water flow.	Clean the filter according to the manufacturer's instructions.
	A pipe is blocked downstream.	Locate and remove the obstruction.
	The piping is too small.	Contact a service technician to replace the piping with properly sized pipe.
	The skimmer and the pump strainer basket are clogged.	Empty and clean the skimmer and the strainer basket.
	The pump impeller and diffuser are clogged or worn.	Clear any obstructions. Contact a service technician to replace worn parts.
	The pump is undersized.	Resize equipment accordingly.
Cycles are shorter than is normal between back-washes.	The water is not balanced and/or the sanitizer residual is too low.	Balance the water and maintain the proper sanitizer residual.
	The flow rate is excessive.	Restrict the flow to the rated capacity of the filter.
	The filter is undersized.	Install a larger filter or an additional filter.
	There's an unusual burden on the filter, caused by excessive dirt, debris, body oil, algae, or other contaminants.	Do your best to keep debris out of the water. Encourage bathers to shower before entering the pool or spa.
	The filter element isn't being cleaned properly.	Follow the manufacturer's guidelines for cleaning and backwashing the filter.
Filtering is poor.	The sanitizer residual is low.	Maintain adequate sanitizer residual.
	The filter is too small, the flow rate is too low, and/or the operating time is too short to obtain an adequate turnover of the water.	Contact a service technician to verify that all equipment is properly sized for your pool or spa.
	The filter isn't being cleaned effectively.	Cartridge filters should be cleaned thoroughly, and DE and sand filters should be backwashed completely.

(chart continues)

Troubleshooting the Filter

PROBLEM	POSSIBLE CAUSES	SOLUTION
Filtering is poor.	The pump is too large.	Reduce the flow rate.
	The filter is installed backward.	Replumb correctly.
Sand or DE is entering the pool.	If you have a sand filter, it may be channeling.	*Channeling* refers to formation of channels in the sand bed, which allow water to pass through unfiltered. Backwash the filter to redistribute the sand. Check the water level to make sure air isn't getting into the system.
	If you have a sand filter, it may have mud balls.	If the filter hasn't been backwashed consistently, mud balls may have formed. Or the sand may have calcified and is no longer able to filter out dirt. Remove the affected sand and replace it with fresh sand. Backwash the filter.
	If you have a DE filter, the DE may have coagulated or solidified.	If you notice hardening of the DE cake, remove the grids and clean the elements, following the manufacturer's instructions. Reassemble the filter and add fresh DE.
	If you have a DE filter, the DE isn't adequately coating the grids.	Make sure the pump and filter are sized accordingly. Make sure the DE slurry isn't being fed into the skimmer too quickly.
	If you have a cartridge filter, its fabric may be torn, allowing unfiltered water to pass through.	Replace the damaged cartridge.
	The backwash valve isn't fully closed.	Close the backwash valve.
	If you have a sand filter, the lateral may be broken.	Replace the broken lateral.
	If you have a DE filter, the fabric on the filter grid may be torn or worn.	Repair any small holes with fingernail polish or silicone sealer. Replace severely damaged filter elements.
Air pressure builds up.	There may be a hairline crack or leak in plumbing connections on the suction side of the pump.	Locate and repair any cracks or leaks. Meanwhile, open the pressure-release valve to allow the air to escape.
	Low water level in the pool is permitting air to enter via the skimmer.	Fill the pool to the proper level. Meanwhile, open the pressure-release valve to allow the air to escape.

Pumps and Motors

s a pool or spa owner, you'll be happy to know that your pump* requires little maintenance so long as it's been installed and operated properly. Nevertheless, the more you know about the pump, the more you'll appreciate it when it's functioning smoothly.

In the first few seconds after a pump is turned on, the shaft accelerates from zero to thousands of rotations per minute. The incredible torque it takes to accomplish this accounts for most of the wear and tear a pump experiences. The pump shaft is connected to the pump's impeller, which subsequently spins, creating a centrifugal force that moves water through the circulation system.

Most pumps are tightly sealed and self-lubricating. They're powered by electricity and should be connected to a ground fault circuit interrupter (GFCI) to prevent accidental electrocution. What differentiates one pump from the next? Let's take a look.

*Note: *Pumps and motors for pools and spas are sold as a single integrated unit, so it's impossible to discuss one without the other. From here on out, when I say* pump, *I mean the combined pump/motor.*

A pool pump and motor are integrated, which is why they're often viewed as a single piece of equipment. With the typical pump and motor, an impeller pulls water through the strainer, which catches large debris, and pumps it on to the filter.

to filter

strainer pot

from pool or spa

motor

volute and impeller

PUMP DESIGN

The more you know about pump design and operation, the more you'll appreciate the difficult task it performs of moving water steadily through your pool and spa filtration system. A basic understanding of pump mechanics will also help you troubleshoot potential problems down the road and maybe even avoid costly service repairs. Here, then, is a quick look at the inner workings of a typical pool and spa pump.

The Motor

Pump motors are available in a wide range of horsepower ratings and with different starter systems and casing materials. All, however, follow the same mechanical principles: A large number of copper wire coils are wound and woven together to form *windings*. The windings take up most of the space inside the cylindrical casing of the motor. A shaft runs through the hollow center of the windings, held in place by bearings at each end of the motor. This shaft carries the armature — an iron and copper electromagnet. When the motor is switched on, an electric current passes through the windings and creates a strong electromagnetic force that turns the armature and shaft at a high speed. The high-speed revolutions of the shaft drive the pump.

Starting the motor, however, is like starting your car — it requires much more energy to start the motor than it does to run it at full speed. To provide this extra boost of electricity, motors have a starting mechanism. Two types are commonly used: switched and switchless.

Switched motors provide an extra boost of electricity when operation of the motor begins. Many switched motors have two compartments; one contains the switch, terminal board, and other sensitive components and the other the windings and bearings. Some experts believe that the two-compartment design separates the "work room" from the "control room" and protects the controls from environmental conditions such as heat and moisture. Switched motors provide a high initial starting torque, which is important if the pump's impeller needs to overcome trapped dust and debris.

Switchless motors store enough of an electric current in a capacitor to start the motor. They use a permanent split capacitor start-and-run design and a continuous duty run capacitor. This design eliminates the use of an internal starting switch and governor, thereby offering greater dependability, according to some experts.

Priming

Most modern swimming pool pumps are self-priming, which means that the pump is always full of water and does not need to be primed with water before starting. Pumps found on older pools may be "regular" pumps (not self-priming). If such a pump loses its prime, the motor can overheat during operation, damaging both the motor and the pump.

The Strainer

A leaf strainer is a standard feature of most pump units sold today. It catches leaves, hair, lint, and other large particles of debris before they can enter and clog the pump. It also holds a reservoir of water that serves to self-prime the pump. Many strainers have a clear, see-through plastic top so you can easily tell whether the basket needs emptying. The strainer should be cleaned regularly. When clogged, it will greatly reduce the flow of water to the filter.

The Impeller

The pump body, or volute, holds the components of the pump, including the impeller. When the impeller spins, water or air is thrown out from the center by its vanes, lowering pressure in the center and creating the pumping action. The depth of the vanes on the impeller determines how much water a pump can move. If you install an impeller with deeper vanes than those of the pump's original vanes, you must also increase the horsepower of the pump.

MAKING REPAIRS

Though the pump and motor are typically sold as a single unit, you may encounter a time when you want to replace just the pump or just the motor. In that case, keep in mind that all the parts need to be properly sized with each other. This includes the mounting face, the shaft, and the horsepower rating, which is determined by the energy draw needed for the impeller.

In some cases, the impeller works in conjunction with a diffuser. The diffuser is a round, flat plate with raised radiating fins. It faces the impeller, with a narrow gap between the two sets of fins or vanes. The diffuser helps the impeller create a vacuum by limiting open space immediately surrounding the impeller. It also promotes water flow through the system. Over a period of time, this diffuser plate can be gouged or worn by tiny bits of gravel or sand that pass through the strainer. Some pumps feature a stainless-steel wear plate to reduce damage to the diffuser.

Occasionally, small stones, grass, and other debris can plug the pump's impeller, impeding the flow of water. If that's the case, disassemble the pump and use a semi-rigid wire to clean the impeller.

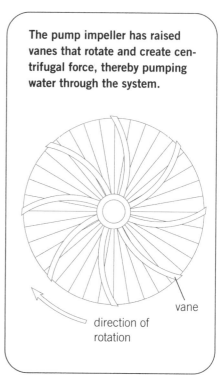

The pump impeller has raised vanes that rotate and create centrifugal force, thereby pumping water through the system.

vane

direction of rotation

The Seal

One other critical component of the pump is the mechanical seal that stops water from leaking out around the shafts between the pump and the electric motor. This mechanical seal is commonly a spring-loaded, rubber-cased unit, which is routinely replaced whenever the pump is professionally disassembled for other repairs. The seal itself uses ceramic and carbon parts. Ceramic and carbon seals are delicate and can be easily cracked if tapped with a screwdriver or other metal object. It's a good idea to know where the seal is and how to identify damage to it. If you determine that it needs to be replaced, call in a pool serviceman; the disassembly of a pump and repair of worn or damaged seals is a job best left to a professional.

SIZING A PUMP CORRECTLY

When sizing a pool pump, bigger isn't always better. A pump that's too large could damage the filter and waste energy, while a pump that's too small may not turn over the water as often as is necessary. To work effectively, a pump must be sized correctly for your pool or spa.

To figure out what size pump you need, you need to know the pool volume in gallons, the flow rate needed to turn over the water (circulate all of the water once through the filtration system) in a certain amount of time, and the system's *total dynamic head* (the flow restriction caused by piping, fittings, and equipment). The builder usually does these calculations when the pool is installed, but it's a good idea to check them again whenever you need to replace a pump just to make sure the calculations are right.

First, calculate the pool capacity using basic geometry (see pages 48–49 for assistance). There are 7.5 gallons of water in 1 cubic foot, so after you've estimated the number of cubic feet in your pool, multiply that number by 7.5 to find the number of gallons the pool can contain.

Next, determine the flow rate needed to circulate that many gallons of water in the specified amount of time. The recommended turnover rate varies by region and among different kinds of pools, but the widely accepted norm is eight hours. Thus, simply divide the number of gallons of water by the turnover time of eight hours to find out how many gallons per hour the pump needs to circulate. You can convert that figure into gallons per minute by dividing by 60. (To convert gallons to liters, multiple the number of gallons by 3.79.)

Finally, total dynamic head (TDH) should be factored into the equation. TDH is the sum of the resistance or friction water encounters as it flows through the circulation system. Pipes, fittings, valves, and equipment cause resistance. For example, the longer a pipe runs and the more turns it makes, the greater the resistance it places on water flowing through it. All components — from the skimmer to main drain — must be accounted for when figuring TDH. If possible, work from a blueprint of the pool's circulation system and list the number of 45-degree elbows, valves, pipes (including their length and size), filters, heaters, and any other equipment attached to the circulation system. Then use the charts provided by pump manufacturers to determine the appropriate *head-loss value* (the amount of pressure, expressed in feet) that each component imposes on the water-circulation system. The total of all the components added together equals the TDH for your pool.

Now you're ready to select a pump that will meet your needs. Most manufacturers provide graphic charts that make it easy to select the proper pump. The chart shows a curve plotted on a grid that indicates the size of pump needed to produce the desired flow rate given the calculated TDH. Simply plot where the flow rate and TDH intersect on the graph, and choose the corresponding pump size. If the plotted point falls between two pumps, choose the larger one.

START-UP

When starting a pump after repair work or after the pump has been off for some time, always make sure the pump contains water. With a self-priming pump, make sure the strainer pot is full of water. Open all suction and discharge valves that may have been closed and bleed the air from the filter tank using the filter's air-release valve before trying to start the pump.

In all other cases, resist the urge to oversize the pump. Your goal is to select the smallest pump possible for the job. If the pump is too large and the flow rate too great, the result could be damaged equipment. If the pump is too small, you won't get adequate filtration.

Also, make sure that the piping can handle the flow rate you want without causing the water to flow too fast. In general, water velocity should not exceed 10 feet per second for discharge piping or 8 feet per second for suction piping, A pool professional can help you determine whether all components are sized properly to work together.

INSTALLING PUMPS

Pool pumps and motors should be installed in a cool, clean, dry location so that dust, leaves, and other debris can't clog the motor's ventilation passages. Don't install a pool pump anywhere near the laundry room. Lint from dryers will be sucked up by the motor fan and clog the air intake. The motor should be covered and slightly elevated so that water puddles will not be sucked into the motor by the cooling fan. Ideally, the motor and pump unit should be enclosed in a waterproof structure with louvered sides to provide ventilation and protection from rain. Some manufacturers will not guarantee motors unless they have been protected in this way.

TWO-SPEED PUMPS

Sometimes, especially in spa applications, two-speed pumps are installed. These can help save energy; the low speed is run during off-peak times to filter the water and the high speed is used to power jets or to accelerate filtration during periods of high bather load. If you opt for a two-speed pump, make sure the low speed pumps enough water for proper filtration.

TROUBLESHOOTING

A pump and motor can fail for a variety of reasons. The following guide looks at some of the most typical problems pool and spa owners encounter. Keep in mind that pump and motor repair can be complicated; don't assume that you should undertake these repairs yourself. In fact, the warranty on the pump may become void if you tamper with the equipment yourself rather than having the work done by an authorized repair professional. If you believe you're qualified to make any of these repairs, proceed with caution. Consult the manufacturer's literature, which often offers its own troubleshooting guide, and be sure to turn off the electrical power before getting to work.

Troubleshooting the Pump

PROBLEM	POSSIBLE CAUSES	SOLUTION
Pump won't run.	The power is turned off at the main supply.	Turn the power on.
	A circuit breaker is tripped or a fuse is blown.	Reset the breaker and/or replace the fuse. If the breaker trips or the fuse blows again, you may have an overloaded circuit, possibly caused by a short circuit in the motor.
	The automatic timer, if you have one, is preventing operation.	Reset the timer or switch to manual operation.
	The motor has overheated.	If the thermal overload switch has been activated, reset it if there is a manual reset button. Keep in mind that something has caused the motor to overheat, such as an obstruction in the inlet. Take the necessary steps to prevent it from happening again.
Pump loses prime.	The pump doesn't have any water in it.	Fill the pump with water and prime again.
	The water level in the pool is low.	Raise the water level to the middle of the skimmer opening to prevent the pump from sucking air.
	A valve in the circulation system is closed.	Open all valves in the circulation system.
	A line is plugged.	Clean the skimmer basket, pump strainer basket, and pump, as necessary.
	The strainer pot lid is not closed tightly.	Check the lid and the O-ring and gasket that seal it. Clean and replace as necessary.
	The suction line has an air leak.	Tighten all pipes and fittings. Locate the leak, if any, and repair.
	The vertical suction lift is too long.	Move the pump so that the vertical lift is no more than 15 feet from the water. A lift of more than 15 feet reduces performance and a lift greater than 25 feet causes loss of prime.
	The flange on the seal is improperly positioned.	Adjust the alignment.
	The seal on the pump is worn.	Check and replace if needed.
	The impeller is out of alignment.	Realign using an impeller gauge.
	The impeller is plugged.	Remove debris and other obstructions.
Pump leaks.	The seal or O-ring is defective.	Replace.
	The strainer lid is damaged.	Replace.

(chart continues)

Troubleshooting the Pump

PROBLEM	POSSIBLE CAUSES	SOLUTION
Water flows too slowly.	The strainer or skimmer basket is full of debris.	Empty the basket.
	The filter is dirty.	Check the filter gauge and backwash or clean the filter as necessary.
	The impeller or diffuser is worn.	Replace.
	The pump is undersized.	Refer to the manufacturer's pump sizing chart to verify that you have the right-size pump. Replace the pump if necessary.
	The vertical suction lift is too long.	Move the pump so that the vertical lift is no more than 15 feet from the water.
Cavitation (air entering the circulation system) occurs.	The inlet piping is undersized.	Make sure the pump and pipe sizes are appropriate for each other. Replace if needed.
	The circulation system is obstructed.	Check the lines on both sides of the pump and remove any obstructions. Check the skimmer and strainer baskets, as well.
Air bubbles in return water.	The pump has an air leak.	Find and repair the leak.
Pump runs slow.	The electric voltage is insufficient.	Use a voltmeter to check the voltage at the motor terminals and at the meter while the pump is running. If the voltage is low, consult the electric company to remedy the situation.
	An electrical connection is loose.	Disconnect the power and tighten loose connections.
Motor hums but won't run.	The impeller is blocked.	Clear debris from impeller area. Hand-spin impeller and motor shaft until it turns freely.
Motor runs but is noisy.	The bearings are worn.	Call a service technician. If you suspect worn bearings, repair immediately, before more damage occurs. Some bearings are fitted with a plastic collar. If the motor is allowed to run with noisy bearings, they will eventually seize, melting the collar. Then the only solution is a new motor.
	The centrifugal switch spring has failed.	Call a service technician.
	The starter winding is burned out.	Call a service technician.
	The motor is rusted or has insufficient lubrication.	Call a service technician.

Pool and Spa Heaters

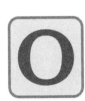ne of the easiest ways to increase the enjoyment of your backyard pool is to heat the water so you can swim comfortably earlier in the spring and later in the fall. In some warm-weather regions, a pool heater can even guarantee pleasant year-round swimming. Of course, with energy costs and conservation always of great concern, it's more important than ever to select an efficient heater that's going to maximize your energy yield.

There are five basic types of pool heaters: gas, electric, oil, heat pump, and solar. The type that's best for you and your pool depends largely on your budget, the cost and availability of various types of energy in your area, the climate where you live, and your preference for one type of heater over another.

GAS HEATERS

In a typical gas heater, water enters via one port and passes through heat exchangers, where the water is heated. The heat exchanger tubes are made of copper, which effectively conducts heat from the burner tray below. After exiting the heat exchangers, the hot water may be mixed with cool pool water as it flows back into the pool.

There are two ignition styles of gas heaters: millivolt (or standing pilot) and electronic pilot. The millivolt heater has

> **CAUTION!**
> Unlike natural gas, propane gas is heavier than air and may settle near the ground if not immediately ignited. To avoid injury from the possible ignition of residual propane, keep your face away from the heater opening when trying to ignite a propane heater.

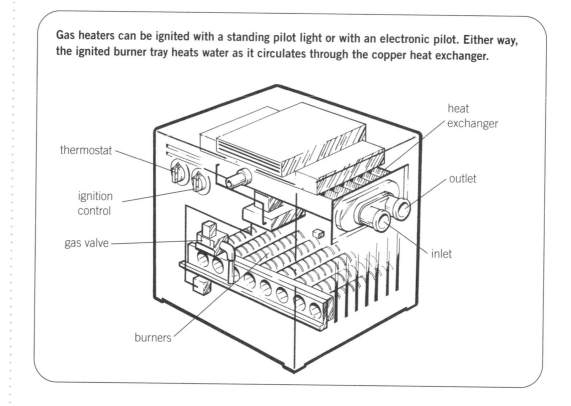

Gas heaters can be ignited with a standing pilot light or with an electronic pilot. Either way, the ignited burner tray heats water as it circulates through the copper heat exchanger.

a pilot light that burns constantly. An electronic pilot heater ignites with an electronic spark. In a millivolt heater, the heat from the pilot light is converted into a small amount of electricity that powers the control circuit, whereas in an electronic pilot heater a small amount of electricity powers the control circuit. Other than the differences in ignition types, these two heaters operate virtually the same way. However, some municipalities permit only electronic pilot ignition, so check with the building authorities or a pool dealer in your area before you buy.

Gas heaters rely on either natural or propane gas for fuel. Most propane gas heaters are made only with millivolt ignition. Traditional gas heaters are shaped like a box, though some models are more egg-shaped.

ELECTRIC HEATERS

An electric heater's components are similar to those of a gas heater, except the heat is generated by an electric coil that either comes in direct contact with the water or wraps around a heat exchanger that transfers heat to the water. The immersed coil is more effective than the heat exchanger, but it's also more vulnerable to the corrosive effects of poorly balanced water. If you have an immersed coil heater and you don't keep your water properly balanced, the heater will eventually fail.

OIL HEATERS

Oil heaters are uncommon, but they can be convenient for those who use oil to heat their home. These units are almost identical in design to gas heaters, except that they burn a special grade of diesel fuel.

HEAT PUMPS

Heat pumps extract heat from the surrounding air and transfer it to pool water. In the typical heat pump, a compressor exerts pressure on a gas, usually Freon, which generates heat. The heat exchanger conducts the heat to the water circulating through the heat pump. The gas cools and is compressed again to generate more heat.

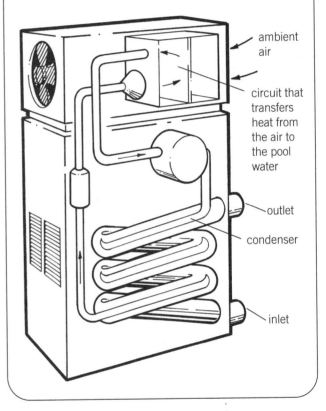

Heat pumps transfer heat from ambient air to the pool water, which is why they work best in warm-weather regions.

ambient air

circuit that transfers heat from the air to the pool water

outlet

condenser

inlet

Because they don't burn fossil fuels, heat pumps are energy efficient and environmentally friendly. They cost 50 to 75 percent less to operate than traditional gas, oil, or electric heaters. However, their initial cost is greater than that of other heater types, and they do have limitations. Because they transfer the heat from the ambient air to the water, heat pumps work best in warm-weather climates. In fact, they're not recommended unless the average daily temperature during the swim season is above 50°F (10°C). They don't make effective spa heaters because they take too long to heat water.

Unlike gas, electric, and oil heaters — which are sized by the amount of Btus (British thermal units) they produce — heat pumps are rated by the ton. A ton is the amount of energy needed to keep one ton of ice at 32°F (0°C) for 24 hours. For the sake of comparison, 1 ton is equal to approximately 15,000 Btus.

SOLAR HEATERS

The solar pool-heating industry has been a veritable hotbed of activity over the past few years. Several factors have prompted this renewed interest in solar heating. The main reason is the rising cost of fossil fuels, especially natural gas. Also fueling interest is the United States' growing alarm regarding our dependence on oil from the Middle East and the reluctance of many Americans to start drilling for domestic oil in some of the nation's most pristine regions.

The science behind solar pool heaters couldn't be simpler. After it runs through the pool's pump and filter, water is diverted to solar collectors. The collectors, made from black polypropylene, are merely panels of tubing through which the water flows. The black polypropylene absorbs the heat of the sun, much like black asphalt in parking lots. As water passes through the collectors, it absorbs heat from the panels before it's returned to the pool.

The water coming into the pool will be a couple of degrees warmer than the pool water, and the entire pool will gradually warm as the water is turned over and over again. Sometimes a separate pump is needed to send the water through the collectors so that the pool's main pump isn't overworked.

Historically, solar heating systems have been a tough sell because they cost more than gas heaters. Whereas a gas heater might go for $2,000, a comparable solar system could cost as much as $3,000 (less in highly competitive markets, such as Florida). However, the rising cost of fossil fuels means that a solar system can more quickly make up that price difference through lower energy bills. Whereas it used to take about five years to start seeing a return on a solar heating system, the rising cost of fossil fuels has shortened that window to just two to three years.

In addition, the solar pool-heating industry has matured and the product has become more reliable. Ten- to 12-year warranties are not uncommon. Plus, the UV inhibitors and stabilizers used in the collectors today are very strong, enabling the solar panels to withstand the brutal sunbaked conditions they're subjected to.

Installing a Solar Heater

Aboveground pools and in-ground pools use different types of solar heaters. The aboveground market is composed mostly of inexpensive cash-and-carry, do-it-yourself products. These units are usually installed on the ground next to the pool. Solar collectors for in-ground pools, on the other hand, are usually mounted on rooftops or hillsides. They can be installed by skilled do-it-yourselfers, but most are installed professionally, especially when automated controls are incorporated or advanced plumbing is required.

Installed under the right conditions, a solar heating system can warm pool water 10 to 15 degrees F (5.6–8.3 degrees C), but it won't perform as well on cloudy or rainy days. (Then again, you're not likely to use the pool in these conditions.)

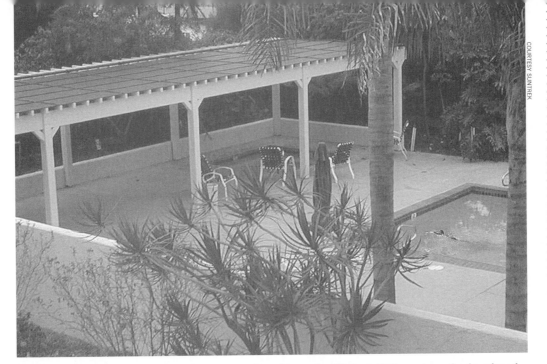

Solar panels can be disguised so they're less obtrusive, as in this installation, where they're placed on top of a poolside arbor.

What is the ideal setup for solar? Though recommendations vary among suppliers, general guidelines for installation, use, and maintenance are as follows:

~ Solar collectors should face south for optimal sun exposure. The panels should get full sun for at least six hours a day. Obviously, the longer the collectors are in full sun, the better they work.

~ The surface area of the collectors should equal at least 50 percent of the pool's surface area. Additional collector surface area will need to be added to compensate for pool water that is shaded or deep, for windy terrain, and for other heat-sapping features. If you want to use your pool year-round, add additional panels for use in the cooler months.

~ If the pool is relatively new, the existing pump is probably sufficient to circulate water through the solar collectors without compromising the effectiveness of the pool's filtration system. In some instances, a larger pump may be needed. If the collectors are cool to the touch when the water is running through them on a warm day, you can rest assured that you're getting enough flow.

~ It's difficult to heat spas with solar heaters because hot tubs are typically used in the evening when the sun isn't shining. However, solar-heated water can be diverted to the spa during the day. Then the spa's gas or electric heater doesn't have to work so hard to bring the temperature up later.

- If a pool is equipped with an automatic chlorinator or other chemical sanitizing device, it's best to plumb the sanitizing unit after the solar panels so that the panels aren't exposed to the harsh chemicals. Likewise, systems that use chlorine tablets in the skimmer could cause the solar collectors to deteriorate prematurely. Also, some experts recommend waiting 48 hours after shocking pool water before routing water through the solar collectors again.
- Turn the solar system off when you're backwashing the filter, and don't turn it back on until the system has run for at least 20 minutes after backwashing. This prevents debris from entering the solar collectors.
- Always cover the pool at night with a solar blanket or pool cover to retain heat, and bypass the solar system at night and during chilly days so that it doesn't cool the water.
- If the pool is not getting warm enough despite ideal solar heating conditions, make sure the filter is not clogged and restricting flow, the timer clock (which tells the circulation system when to divert water through the solar panels) is set for the best times of day, the thermostat on automatic systems isn't set too low, the diverter valve isn't misdirected, the pump isn't too weak to pump the required volume of water, and a sufficient number of collectors are being used for the type of pool being heated.
- Like other pool equipment, solar collectors must be completely drained when winterizing a pool to avoid freeze damage.

Solar Aesthetics

Despite the growing demand for solar pool heaters, aesthetic issues are enough to keep many consumers from purchasing them. After all, a roll of black tubing atop one's roof isn't the most attractive architectural feature of a home.

To address the design issue, some manufacturers have devised systems that reduce the number of brackets and other hardware necessary to secure the panels to the roof. Another design technique is to incorporate a flat roof over a covered patio area and place the solar collectors there. Though black panels collect more solar energy than any other color of panel, some manufacturers offer terra-cotta-colored collectors that blend with the terra-cotta roofs popular in parts of the South and West. Though the terra-cotta collectors are 12 to 30 percent less efficient than black ones, some owners are willing to opt for the less efficient collectors if they will yield a more attractive installation.

If a solar heating system is going to be installed during new construction, certain design steps can downplay the presence of the solar collectors. For example, if the shingles on the roof of the house are black, they'll blend well

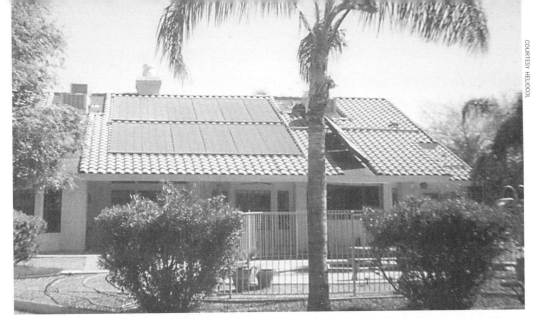
Most solar collector panels are installed on rooftops. Though black collectors would be more effective, here terra-cotta-colored panels blend in with the roof.

with the black solar collectors. If a poolhouse is part of the project, it can be positioned so that the back faces south and the solar collectors can be placed on its roof, completely out of view.

The Benefits of Solar

Though the debate over aesthetics could go on forever, one fact is indisputable: Pools are one of the most inefficient means of storing energy. Whereas lawn mowers and chain saws use a tremendous amount of energy, they are seen as providing a significant use for the energy they consume. Pools heated with fossil fuels, on the other hand, are not seen as providing a benefit in proportion to the energy they consume.

The U.S. Department of Energy has been a longtime supporter of solar energy for heating pools. The Canadian government, meanwhile, recently finished a five-year study on solar energy and strongly recommends the use of solar as a way to reduce greenhouse gases. In fact, the study estimates that if 30 percent of Canadian pool owners converted to solar heating, greenhouse gases would be cut by 280,000 tons over the next 20 years.

SIZING A HEATER CORRECTLY

If you're going to invest in a pool heater, you'll want one that's sized correctly for your particular setup. It must be able to heat the pool water to the desired temperature in the desired amount of time. An undersized heater will heat too slowly. An oversized heater will do the job, but you'll end up spending more for the unit than you have to.

Surface Area and Volume

To select the right-size heater for your pool or spa, you must determine how much water you're trying to heat. For a pool, you'll also need to know how large the surface area is, because most of the water's heat is lost through the surface of the water. That's why one of the best ways to conserve heat in a swimming pool is to cover it when it's not in use. For a spa, which is covered with an insulating cover when it's not in use, surface area is less important than total volume. To determine the surface area, use one of these formulas:

~ **Rectangle or square:** length x width
~ **Circle:** ½ the diameter x ½ the diameter x 3.14
~ **Oval:** ½ the length x ½ the width x 3.14
~ **Kidney:** length x width x 0.75
~ **Free-form:** Break the pool into smaller geometric shapes, determine their area, and add all the areas together.

To convert square feet into square meters, if needed, multiply by 0.0929. To calculate the volume, determine the surface area using the guidelines above and multiply by the average depth. This will give you a fairly accurate cubic-foot measurement of the water volume. To determine the number of gallons, multiply the cubic footage by 7.5 (the number of gallons in a cubic foot). To convert gallons to liters, if needed, multiply by 3.79.

Wind Velocity

Wind promotes evaporation, which is the main source of heat loss in swimming pools. Therefore, take note of the average wind velocity in your area, an important factor when determining heater size. Man-made or natural windbreaks around the pool can cut down on heat loss due to wind.

To determine wind velocity, you can check with the National Weather Service in your area, or you can simply watch the weather report during local news broadcasts and note the wind speed on what feels like a typical day.

When and How to Heat

You'll also want to look at how you plan to use your pool to determine whether you'll need to heat it continually (all the time) or intermittently (only when needed). If you swim in your pool almost daily, you'll want to maintain the temperature at a set point; if you swim only on weekends, you'll want to heat the water only for those times. Continual heating requires a unit that can compensate for heat loss at the surface of the pool or spa, whereas intermittent heating requires a unit that can heat the total volume of water in a specified amount of time. It takes a lot more energy to raise the temperature of water several degrees than it does to maintain the higher temperature, but this cost may still be less than the cost to maintain a certain temperature at all times. Though everyone's pool use differs somewhat, a general rule of thumb is to turn off the heater if your pool won't be used for three days or more.

Continual Heating

For continual heating, the main factor in determining heater size is how much of a temperature rise you want to maintain. The recommended range for swimming is 78 to 82°F (26–28°C). For spas, 104°F (40°C) is the maximum temperature recommended.

After you know what temperature you want to achieve, then determine the average daily temperature for the coldest month you'll be heating your pool or spa. If you plan to keep your pool open year-round, the coldest month might be January or February; for the traditional swimming season, it's more likely to be May or September. By subtracting this average daily temperature from the desired temperature you want for swimming or soaking, you can calculate the needed rise in temperature.

Heater manufacturers and pool dealers can provide you with charts that will help you determine how many Btus your heater will need to generate to achieve the temperature rise you need. Below is an example of one based on a wind velocity of 3.5 mph. A series of formulas is also typically provided to allow you to convert to other wind velocities, say 5 or 10 mph.

Sizing a Heater for Continual Heating

	TEMPERATURE RISE NEEDED				
	10°F (5.6°C)	15°F (8.3°C)	20°F (11.1°C)	25°F (13.9°C)	30°F (16.7°C)
SURFACE AREA	REQUIRED HEATER OUTPUT (BTUS PER HOUR)				
200 sq. ft. (18.6 m²)	21,000	31,500	42,000	52,500	63,000
300 sq ft. (27.9 m²)	31,500	47,300	73,000	78,800	94,500
400 sq. ft. (37.2 m²)	42,000	63,000	84,000	105,000	126,000
500 sq. ft. (46.5 m²)	52,500	78,800	105,000	131,000	157,000
600 sq. ft. (55.7 m²)	63,000	94,500	126,000	157,000	189,000
700 sq. ft. (65 m²)	73,500	110,000	147,000	184,000	220,000
800 sq. ft. (74.3 m²)	84,000	126,000	168,000	210,000	252,000
900 sq. ft. (83.6 m²)	94,500	142,000	189,000	236,000	284,000
1,000 sq. ft. (92.9 m²)	105,000	157,000	210,000	263,000	315,000

Let's assume you have a pool with a 700-square-foot surface area, the wind speed is 3.5 mph, the average daily temperature for the coldest month you plan to swim is 55 degrees, and you'd like the pool water to be 78 degrees. By subtracting 55 from 78, you see that you need a temperature rise of 23 degrees. Looking at the columns for a 20-degree rise and a 25-degree rise, you can see that to maintain the 23-degree rise you want for a surface area of 700 square feet, you'll need a heater that can produce between 147,000 and 184,000 Btus per hour.

Intermittent Heating

If you want to heat the pool only intermittently, the total volume of water is more important than surface area. For pools, the heater should be able to heat the water to the desired temperature within 24 hours. For spas, the heater should be able to heat the water within 30 minutes.

Using volume as the deciding factor, here is a typical heater-sizing chart for a spa using an intermittent-style gas heater to achieve a rise in temperature of 30 degrees F (17 degrees C).

Sizing a Chart for Intermittent Heating

| SPA VOLUME | HEATER INPUT (BTUS PER HOUR) | | | | |
| | 125,000 | 175,000 | 250,000 | 325,000 | 400,000 |
	MINUTES REQUIRED FOR A 30-DEGREE RISE IN TEMPERATURE				
200 gallons (757 L)	30	21	15	12	9
300 gallons (1,136 L)	45	32	23	17	14
400 gallons (1,514 L)	60	43	30	23	19
500 gallons (1,893 L)	75	54	38	29	23
600 gallons (2,271 L)	90	64	45	35	28
700 gallons (2,650 L)	105	75	53	40	33
800 gallons (3,028 L)	120	86	60	46	37
900 gallons (3,407 L)	135	96	68	52	42
1,000 gallons (3,785 L)	150	107	75	58	47

The Magic Formula

Heating charts like the ones on pages 107 and 108 are available from heater manufacturers, making the task of selecting the right heater as simple as plotting points on a graph. If you want to size a heater without the convenience of one of these charts, you can use this basic formula:

Gallons x 8.33 x temperature rise in degrees Fahrenheit = Btus required

In this formula, 8.33 represents the number of pounds in a gallon of water. If you have a 40,000-gallon pool and you needed a 15-degree temperature rise, your equation would read: 40,000 x 8.33 x 15 = 4,998,000 Btus. You can divide 4,998,000 by the desired heat-up time to determine the number of Btus needed per hour. If you want the pool to be heated in 24 hours, simply divide 4,998,000 by 24 to determine that you need a heater with an output of 208,250 Btus per hour.

Other Variables

Sizing a heater isn't simply about numbers, however. You also need to consider the pool and spa's location and what type of environmental elements they're exposed to. Wind, especially, causes excessive heat loss. If your pool is frequently exposed to windy conditions (defined as winds over 10 mph), you may need to increase your heater size by as much as 25 percent. You can greatly reduce the impact of wind on your heating costs by constructing a wind barrier, such as a fence or natural wall of evergreen shrubs and trees.

Also, a pool that's mostly in the shade and doesn't absorb any energy from the sun may require a larger heater, and pools in high altitudes should also increase their heater size. A pool professional can look at your particular situation and make an informed recommendation.

TROUBLESHOOTING

Heaters should be installed and serviced by trained professionals to make sure they're in proper working order. That said, take a look at some of the most common heating-related problems on page 110. You may be able to take care of some of these yourself; others will require a call to a service technician.

Troubleshooting a Heater

PROBLEM	POSSIBLE CAUSES	SOLUTION
Heater won't heat water to desired temperature.	The heater isn't running long enough.	Adjust the time clock.
	The filter is dirty.	Clean or backwash the filter.
	The thermostat is faulty.	Replace as needed.
	The pressure switch is damaged.	Replace as needed.
	The heater is undersized.	Upsize heater as needed.
	If you have a gas heater, the gas supply is insufficient.	Check the piping and gas-supply system to make sure it's sized properly.
Soot has formed in the combustion chamber of a gas or oil heater.	Water is flowing too quickly through the heater.	Adjust the flow and clean the heat exchanger.
	The air supply is inadequate.	Check for proper installation and venting, especially on indoor installations.
	The air inlet or venturi is plugged.	Check for dirt and debris and clean it out.
Heater isn't running long enough to heat the water.	The timer is malfunctioning.	Adjust the timer and clean the exchanger.
	If you have a gas heater, the gas valve regulator needs adjustment.	Adjust as needed.
Heater switches on and off repeatedly.	The filter is dirty.	Clean or backwash the filter.
	The water level is low.	Raise the water to proper level.
	The manual bypass needs adjustment.	Adjust the bypass.
	The pressure switch is broken.	Adjust or repair the switch so the heater shuts off when the pump shuts off.
Scale forms in the heat exchanger.	The water is not balanced.	Bring total alkalinity, pH, and calcium hardness within acceptable levels.
Heat exchanger is corroding.	The water is acidic.	Balance the water.
Burner flame is weak.	If you have a gas heater, the gas pressure is low.	Check gas pipe and meter sizes and/or adjust the gas pressure.
	Dirt and debris are plugging the burners.	Clean the burners.
The heater knocks or whines.	The heater is operating after the pump shuts off.	Adjust or replace the pressure switch.
	Something is blocking the system.	Remove the blockage and flush the system.
	Scale has built up in the heat exchanger.	Clean or replace the heat exchanger.
	The pressure switch is out of adjustment.	Adjust the pressure switch.

ENERGY CONSERVATION TIPS

The following tips come from the U.S. Department of Energy and can help you reduce your pool heating costs.

1. Keep a thermometer in your pool. It will help you determine the temperature that is perfect for you.

2. Keep your pool thermostat at the lowest setting that will maintain a comfortable swimming environment.

3. Mark the "comfort setting" on the thermostat dial to avoid accidental or careless overheating.

4. Lower your thermostat setting to 70°F (21°C) when the pool isn't going to be used for three or four days. For longer periods, shut the pool heater off.

5. Use a fence or hedge as a windbreak to protect your pool from wind-related heat loss. A 7 mph (2.6 kph) wind at the surface of the pool can triple a pool's heat loss.

6. Use a pool cover when the pool is not in use. A cover can reduce your pool's energy consumption by 50 to 75 percent.

7. Get your pool heater tuned up annually. A properly tuned pool heater will operate more efficiently.

For more information about all types of pool heaters, visit the Department of Energy Web site at www.energy.gov.

Pool and Spa Covers

Covering your pool or spa when it's not in use is smart for a number of reasons. A cover helps safeguard the water when adults aren't present to supervise. It also reduces evaporation, lowers heating costs, helps keep the water clean, and reduces the rate at which sanitizers dissipate in the water. Any one of these reasons should convince you of the need to cover your pool or spa.

POOL COVERS

Covers for aboveground pools are usually designed for winterizing. These types of covers are little more than massive tarps that can be tied down over the pool walls. A cover for an in-ground pool, on the other hand, may be available in a range of options, depending on how the cover will be used. Some in-ground-pool covers are designed primarily for winterizing, while others are supposed to be pulled out whenever the pool is not being used or is left unsupervised. Many in-ground-pool covers are integrated into the pool design so that they virtually disappear when not in use.

Innovative manufacturing techniques now enable homeowners to order a pool cover to fit almost any pool configuration — from multilevel geometric pools to curvaceous free-form creations. And pool builders — once concerned that any mention of safety would send a prospective pool buyer running for the door — now realize that they have a *better* chance of making the sale if they address a buyer's safety concerns head-on. Combined, these trends have boosted the popularity of pool covers to an all-time high.

Though there are a lot of similarities among the in-ground pool covers offered by the top manufacturers, there are also some significant differences in design and construction that make it worth your time to comparison shop. To ensure you're purchasing the in-ground pool cover that best meets your needs, consider the following issues.

Track versus Tie-Down

Though the difference between the two may be an elementary concept for pool owners, aspiring pool owners will want to consider the pros and cons of these two broad categories of safety covers before deciding which one to purchase.

Track covers. These covers are composed of a roll of vinyl stored on a reel system and attached to tracks that run the length of the pool. They are available in two versions: manual and automatic. The manual version requires that someone physically crank the cover open and pull it shut, whereas the automatic version uses a motorized system to accomplish these tasks. At least one company has partially automated its manual cover by incorporating a system that uses a cordless drill to drive the cover mechanism. The track design, whether manual or automatic, makes these covers convenient for everyday use.

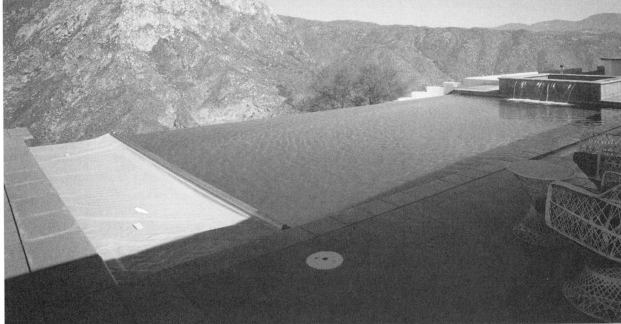

Automatic pool covers are versatile enough to fit most any pool design, including this vanishing-edge pool.

Tie-down covers. This family of pool covers secures the pool with a sheet of vinyl or mesh that's been reinforced with stitched webbing. The cover is installed using springs and adjustable straps that attach to deck-mounted anchors. These covers can be quite heavy and are installed mainly by pool professionals as part of the process of winterizing a pool. They are too cumbersome for day-to-day use.

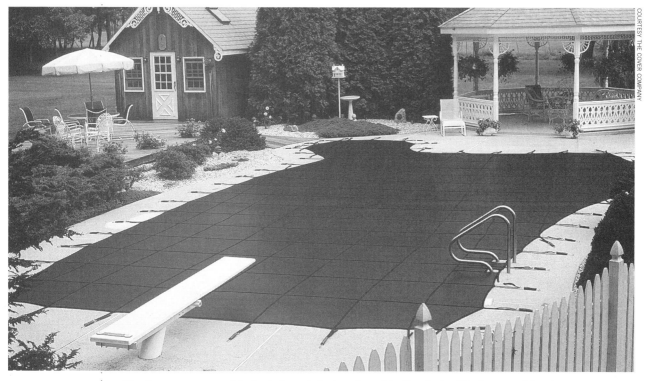

Tie-down covers consist of reinforced vinyl anchored to the deck with straps and hardware.

Material Matters

Just like the pools they cover, not all pool covers are created equal. And differences in materials and manufacturing can make the difference between a cover that fails after a couple of seasons and one that continues to perform for many years. Indeed, materials play a significant role in a cover's overall quality.

Your first area of scrutiny for a new cover, whether a tie-down or a track cover, is the thickness of the vinyl. Most manufacturers use a 10- to 14-ounce vinyl; the heavier the vinyl, the thicker it is. A heavier vinyl may be more resistant to punctures and scuffs, but it also will be more cumbersome to work with.

Is the vinyl coated or laminated? Laminated vinyl is composed of a scrim (an open-weave fabric) glued between two pieces of vinyl. In coated vinyl, on the other hand, the scrim is incorporated while the vinyl is still in its liquid form, making it unnecessary to glue the pieces together. A laminated vinyl is prone to shrinkage; your pool supply company will need to accommodate for this shrinkage when the cover is sized. Other than the shrinkage issue, both types of vinyl perform well.

Both laminated and coated vinyl covers should be treated with UV protectors on the topside and algae preventives on the bottom side. Mildew inhibitors and colorfast treatments are also beneficial; some covers have them, while others don't. Some suppliers argue that whether the cover is laminated or coated is less important than the ingredients — such as UV protectors and mildew inhibitors — that go into the vinyl.

Tie-down covers have, in addition to vinyl, a number of material components that must be examined carefully. Note the differences among the covers you're considering in terms of the following:

Webbing. Some manufacturers of tie-down covers stitch webbing only on the top and the first couple feet of the underside, while others stitch webbing on the entire top and bottom. Double webbing can make the cover sturdier. However, a cover's integrity also depends on the quality of the mesh or vinyl being used, the weight of the vinyl, and how closely together the webbing is sewn.

Stitching. A well-crafted tie-down cover shouldn't have any loose, missed, or unfinished stitching. Such flaws may not affect a cover's performance during the first couple of years, but they can lead to cover failure down the road. Some suppliers stitch the vinyl with a thread in a contrasting color so it's easier to see and correct errors.

Anchors, springs, and straps. These items vary slightly among manufacturers. All springs will be made of stainless steel to weather the elements, but their weight and gauge may vary. Though bigger isn't necessarily better, you do want to make sure you're getting the quality necessary for your particular pool. For example, larger-gauge springs may be necessary in areas with heavy snow loads.

Installation tool. The stainless-steel rod used to attach tie-down straps to their anchors varies primarily in length. The only advantage to the longer tool is that the installer doesn't have to lean over as far to slip the grommet over the anchor.

Edging material. If you're going to place a tie-down cover over a pool with rock waterfalls or other irregular outcroppings, you'll need one with flexible edging material sewn to that section of the cover to ensure a snug fit. Edging material differs somewhat among suppliers and you might find one more to your liking than the others. Some manufacturers use a step-cut sewing process that enables covers to go up and over raised walls.

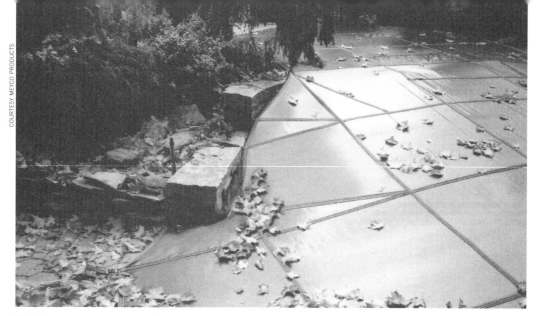

Tie-down covers can be designed to fit securely around most any obstacle, including a rock wall.

Despite all of these differences among pool cover components, it's important to judge a cover's quality by looking at the whole product, not just the individual parts. If you examine only a particular component — like vinyl — you're not getting a full picture of the product. Plus, the best materials in the world won't make a superior pool cover unless the manufacturer knows the best way to assemble them. It's the care and detail in the manufacturing process that matters, and that's what you should look for. All covers have basic materials in common, but what makes the difference is how those materials are fabricated to make a cover that's going to fit properly and last.

Check out the warranties that different manufacturers offer, and read the fine print. In a broad sense, manufacturers that offer a better warranty are more confident of the performance of their product.

Power Performance

With a track system cover, you'll want to examine the gear mechanism that will power the cover over the track.

Manual covers. Manual systems work best for smaller pools because they can require a lot of arm power to operate. Before purchasing one, check out for yourself how it feels to crank the cover open or pull it across the pool. If you find a cover difficult to open and close, you're not likely to use it all the time — negating its use as a true safety cover. Some pool builders may have manual covers on their display pools that you can test out. If not, ask to visit the pools of a few of their customers so you can see the cover in operation firsthand and even try it out.

Automatic covers. Most automatic pool covers use clutch motors that shift into one gear to open the cover and another to close it. A far cry from the loud, unwieldy motors used 30 years ago, today's motors have steel gears and oil-impregnated bearings so the unit doesn't have to be greased periodically. At least one company uses a dual hydraulic motor system; one motor extends the cover and the other retracts it, thus eliminating the clutch system altogether.

Make sure that the motor casing is waterproof. This way, if the recessed vault — where the cover and reel system are stored — ever floods, the drive system won't be damaged. A waterproof motor is also essential in areas where the climate is humid and corrosive.

You'll also want to check your control options. Some covers can be operated only with a key at the pool. Pricier but more convenient models offer in-home control panels and remote control options. After all, when the doorbell rings while you're poolside, you'll be more likely to properly close the pool before answering the door if the controls are convenient.

Fine Design for Track Covers

Not so many years ago, pools with retractable pool covers could be identified by telltale signs: two parallel strips of tracking along the deck and a cover reel system looming at one end of the pool. Today's track-system covers are more likely to be incorporated into the pool's structural design to make them as invisible as possible.

Unless your pool is a simple rectangle, you'll need to custom-order a track cover. If you're building a new pool, make sure your builder is familiar with the cover options available and the installation requirements for your pool design

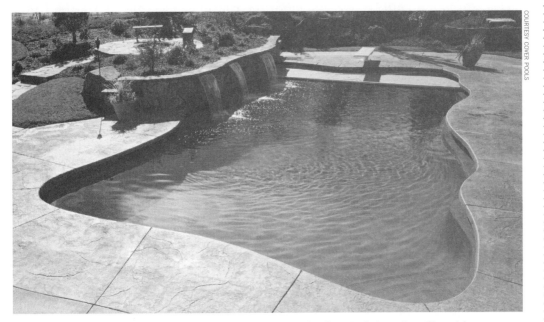

COURTESY COVER POOLS

Under-track systems keep this automatic pool cover completely out of view when it's not in use.

so that you can figure out a way to disguise the cover. If you're retrofitting a pool with a track-system cover, see if you can get colored tracks that blend with your pool deck. Other design elements to consider include the following:

Recessed covers. If you're like many homeowners, you're concerned about how well your pool blends with your home, landscaping, and outdoor furnishings — and the last thing you want to see is evidence of an unsightly pool cover. For this reason, many automatic pool covers are installed below deck level with under-track systems. The lid over the reel's vault can be painted to help it blend in with the decking. Some manufacturers offer lids that can be covered with the same decking material as the rest of the pool for a truly seamless look.

Encapsulated tracks. Encapsulated tracks include a track not only for the cover, but also for the vinyl-liner bead if it's for a vinyl-lined pool and a channel for perimeter fiber-optic lighting. Some manufacturers offer more options and combinations of tracks than others, so make sure your dealer carries the variety you'll need for the type of pool you're building.

Colors. Look for a supplier that offers a variety of color choices — for both the cover fabric as well as the hardware that shows. Then you can pick the cover system that blends with the rest of the pool, the landscape, and your home.

Convertibility. If you purchase a manual track cover, you may wish to look for one that is easily convertible to an automatic cover. Most manual track covers can be converted to automatic covers, but some convert more easily than others. If you ever decide to upgrade, you'll want the service call to be quick and painless, and you won't want the upgrade to be costly. You can expect to pay about 10 percent more for the upgrade than if you had purchased the automatic cover in the first place.

Dealer Support

The best product doesn't always equate with the best supplier. That's why it's important to check out each company's record on support issues. Even the best pool cover won't perform well if it's installed improperly. So make sure your dealer knows what he or she is doing. Ask to see other pools with covers he or she has installed so that you can check with their owners and ask how well they're operating. As with most any purchase, if you buy from a dealer who is knowledgeable and skilled, you'll be happy. It's that simple.

SPA COVERS

Insulated spa covers are crucial to hot tub enjoyment. By keeping heat in the spa and dirt and debris out, these covers help ensure that the tub is ready whenever you are. Most spa covers consist of a foam core covered with vinyl — but not all spa covers are created equal. The type of materials used, the method of construction, and the product design all play a role in whether a cover will prematurely sag, break, or become waterlogged. Under normal wear and tear, the cheapest of covers should last a couple of years, but high-quality covers can last more than five years before showing signs of deterioration.

What makes one spa cover better than the rest? Let's look at the factors that differentiate one spa cover from the next:

Foam Core

Usually made of expanded polystyrene, the foam core is the insulation in an insulated spa cover. The greater the foam density, the stronger the cover will be and the more insulation it will provide. Most spas contain foam with a 1-, 1.5-, or 2-pound (0.45, 0.68, or 0.91 kg) density, which equates to how much 1 cubic foot of the material weighs. Keep in mind that a cover with a greater density weighs more overall, making it harder to move than a lighter-weight cover. This could be important if you don't have a cover-removal device (see page 121) and aren't strong enough to move the heavier cover easily. Convenience aside, you may need the heavier cover if you live in an area where it snows heavily or the winds are high.

Reinforcement

In many insulated spa covers, the foam core is reinforced with aluminum and/or steel supports. These supports typically run along the thick end of the core that meets in the center, where the two sides hinge together. Though there are different styles of reinforcement, the most important thing is that your cover has some.

Taper

Most spa covers are tapered so that rain and melting snow can easily run off the cover and not pool on the surface. Some spa covers have a 4-to-2-inch (10 to 5 cm) taper, which means that they're 4 inches (10 cm) thick in the center and taper to 2 inches (5 cm) thick on the sides. For greater durability, some companies make covers with a 3½-to-2½-inch (9 to 6 cm) taper.

Moisture Barrier

Over time, water will seep through the vinyl exterior of the cover. If the foam core inside the vinyl is allowed to become waterlogged, the additional weight can make the cover sag and break. It may become so heavy that it's difficult to move and puts excessive strain on any cover-removal device you may have.

Plus, a misshapen, waterlogged cover can no longer insulate the spa as well as it should. As a result, the spa loses heat at an incredibly energy-inefficient rate. To prevent — or at least impede — this from happening, choose a spa cover in which the foam core is covered with a vapor barrier.

A vapor barrier is a plastic film that surrounds the core to keep moisture out. Keep in mind, however, that not all plastics are equally effective at resisting moisture. Ask your dealer what the vapor barrier's "vapor transmission coefficient" is. A 0 is ideal, but only a few materials — among them Saran Wrap — can achieve that rating. Anything slightly over 0 is acceptable, however.

The vapor barrier must also be sealed properly or it will be useless. Even a tiny hole or gap can allow moisture in to destroy the core. Three methods of sealing are heat sealing, shrink wrapping, and taping. Any of these methods is acceptable. The important part is that a vapor barrier exists; otherwise, the foam core will quickly become waterlogged.

Vinyl

The foam core is surrounded by vinyl — one type for the underside and another for the topside and skirt. Topside vinyl doesn't offer much in terms of comparing quality among different spa covers. In general, just be sure that you have a marine-grade vinyl with UV inhibitors and a topcoat that will resist abrasions and hold in the color. Then turn your scrutiny to underside vinyl. For the underside, many suppliers use a solid vinyl that better resists steam and chemicals than a lower-quality material. Because water will find its way into the cover no matter how it's constructed, it's important that the underside of the cover have grommets or drainage holes built into it to enable trapped moisture to escape.

Also check how vinyl pieces are sewn together. Too many stitches per inch can weaken the vinyl, while too few won't provide enough support. A good amount is five or six per inch. Make sure all stress points are reinforced and that the stitching won't unravel if accidentally cut. Quality stitching ensures that the cover will retain as much heat as possible, especially at the hinge area.

Skirt

The vinyl flap that hangs from the cover is called the skirt. This material is crucial for keeping wind out of the spa and trapping heat in. The length of the skirt depends on the type of spa you have and how it's been installed. For example, a freestanding spa with a tall lip may benefit from a skirt that's 3 inches (8 cm) or more. If the spa is sunk below ground or recessed in a deck, however, a shorter skirt that stops just short of the ground or deck is recommended.

CAUTION!

Tie-downs are used to lock the spa cover when it's closed. Don't open or close the cover by pulling on these straps or they'll wear prematurely.

Tie-Downs and Handles

Make sure tie-down straps and handles are stitched securely to the cover. These items are stressed every time the cover is used, so they need to be constructed of quality materials that can withstand lots of use. Insert your hand through the handles to make sure they fit adequately, especially if you have large fingers. Also scrutinize the locking hardware to make sure it's sturdy and capable of doing its job of keeping unsupervised children and uninvited guests out of the spa.

Spa Cover Care

Over time, the topside vinyl on a spa cover can dry out and crack. To extend the life of your spa cover, you should clean it and condition it every few months or whenever it looks particularly dirty. Special cleaners and conditioners are available at most spa supply stores. Be sure to clean the underside of the cover, too, as bacteria, mold, and algae can reside there. You may need to use a disinfectant (such as Lysol) to remove mold and mildew odors.

If the foam core has absorbed water, making your 40-pound (18 kg) cover weigh closer to 100 pounds (45 kg), try to dry it out. You can unzip the vinyl jacket on most covers and remove the foam core for air drying. If there's a plastic seal around the foam core, don't attempt to unwrap it unless your cover is so waterlogged that your only other option is to buy a new one. Then you're really not risking anything by unwrapping the plastic from around the core so it can dry out. After the core has dried, you can attempt to rewrap it in plastic, keeping the seams up away from the water surface and using duct tape to seal all seams before reinserting the foam core back into the vinyl jacket.

Spa Cover–Removal Devices

Automatic and manual pool covers have a removal mechanism built right into the unit, but spa covers don't. Fortunately, a new spa cover is light enough that it can easily be moved by hand. However, after it begins to absorb water, the cover can become too heavy for some spa users to remove with ease. That's when some people simply fold open half of their spa cover and enjoy only the exposed portion, rather than struggling to remove the entire cover.

Fortunately, there's a host of spa cover–removal devices on the market to make the job of removing and replacing a spa cover as easy as turning on the spa jets. A cover-removal device also helps you properly store the cover so that it doesn't rest on the ground, where it can become distorted or punctured.

Basically, all cover-removal systems simplify the handling of the cover. Beyond that, they break down into three general types:

~ Low-end units composed of wood or metal support arms at the lip of the spa. The arms may or may not be retractable. You fold the spa cover and push it onto these support arms. To replace the cover, you simply push it back over the spa. These units require a lot of clearance — the width of a folded cover — and offer no mechanical assistance, except that the cover doesn't need to be lifted off the ground to be replaced.

~ Units made of steel or aluminum that mount to the spa cabinet's rear or sides. The cover is folded over a support bar, from which the cover hangs as it is pulled or pushed behind the spa. These units typically offer gas spring assistance and require up to 2 feet (0.6 m) of clearance.

~ Units made of steel or aluminum that mount to the top of a spa cabinet or deck. The cover is folded over a support bar, from which the cover hangs as it is lifted to an upright position, creating a wall or privacy screen. These units typically offer locking gas spring assistance, so they won't blow over in the wind, and require practically no clearance.

Within each type there are further differences worth noting. For example, some systems attach directly to the cover, thereby reducing wear and tear on the cover's vinyl hinge. Aesthetically speaking, some units are more visually appealing than others. Some basic wood units tie in nicely with spa skirts, and powder coating on several metal units gives them a finished look.

In the end, a cover-removal device will make life easier for you and encourage you to use your spa more often. And anything that entices you to use your hot tub more often is worth consideration.

An insulating spa cover is a "must have" for maintaining a hot tub's high temperature. Spa cover–removal devices are available in many designs and configurations to accommodate most any spa installation.

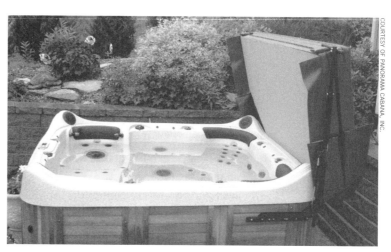

Pool and Spa Automation

ith the exception of landscape lighting, the home automation industry has paid little attention to the backyard. Yet as more homeowners look to convert their exterior space into veritable living rooms, the opportunities for automation are tremendous, especially in the area of hot tubs and swimming pools.

Pools and spas are ideal candidates for automation because they require a great deal of routine maintenance and oversight. In fact, the pool and spa industry has long realized that the major deterrent to sales is the perception that pools and spas are difficult and costly to maintain. If many of the tasks associated with ownership of a pool or spa could be automated, however, more consumers would be likely to consider purchasing one.

Several pool and spa manufacturers understand this reasoning and have made great strides to automate equipment and provide in-home control units for monitoring a pool and spa's performance. Today, pool and spa automation allows homeowners to:

~ Schedule filter cycles to take advantage of off-peak electrical rates
~ Check water temperature and turn the heater on and off accordingly
~ Control pool and landscape lighting
~ Control water features and jets
~ Schedule automatic pool cleaners
~ Guard against frost damage
~ Control the pool and spa from a touch-tone phone
~ Maintain the proper water level
~ Diagnose the most common pool and spa problems from the convenience of an in-home control panel
~ Control the pool or spa with handheld remote controls or wireless devices

Pool and spa automation can be divided into three categories based on how the control signal is sent from the user to the equipment. These are hardwired digital systems, radio frequency systems, and power line carrier systems. Here's a brief explanation of each type.

HARDWIRED SYSTEMS

Hardwired systems have been the most common control system used for pool and spa automation. As the name implies, these systems work by transmitting signals along low-voltage wires installed between a control panel, a command center, and the equipment being controlled. They can be as simple as remote on/off switches and mechanical timers or as elaborate as total control packages that handle underwater and landscape lighting, motorized valves for water features and solar heating systems, and myriad other pool and spa features.

CYBER CONTROL

Not surprisingly, Web-based control of pool and spa functions is the next hurdle for the pool automation industry, with endless opportunities predicted for the new technology. The Internet could provide homeowners with the convenience of controlling their backyard paradise from anywhere in the world. But do you really need that kind of absolute control? Though it would be nice to be able to access your spa control panel from your computer at work and fire up the spa so it's ready by the time you get home, it wouldn't take more than 30 minutes — just enough time to check your messages, get the mail, fix a drink, and shed your clothes — for the spa to warm up after you got home to turn it on yourself. For most people, the ultra-convenience of Web-based control isn't of great value.

The benefits of Web-based pool and spa control seem to be greater for pool and spa service companies than they are for homeowners. Imagine, for example, that you've hired a pool service company with 1,000 pools on its route. A Web interface with these pools would enable the service company to monitor the equipment and troubleshoot problems before driving out to your house. In fact, service technicians could even reprogram pool and spa systems without leaving the office. Your service company could monitor your pool and spa 24 hours a day, 7 days a week, and even program certain information — such as chemical readings and system diagnostics — to be e-mailed to the company monitoring system on a daily basis.

RADIO FREQUENCY SYSTEMS

Radio frequency or RF systems are gaining popularity because of the benefits associated with wireless communications. These systems typically consist of a main control box that sits near a subpanel through which all the equipment is wired. Nothing needs to be wired to the house. Rather, remote control is possible by using handheld, wall-mounted, or portable tabletop remotes.

As an aftermarket product, pool and spa automation has never really taken off because of the hassle of hardwiring controls after a home has been built and all the landscaping has been installed. Understandably, few home-owners want to destroy thousands of dollars' worth of landscaping to install an automation system that could cost them another few thousand dollars. Wireless technology, how-ever, eliminates the need in many instances to disrupt the landscape.

Though reliable wireless systems are new to the pool and spa automation industry, some experts predict that most pool and spa con-trols will be wireless in the future. With no in-home wiring and no need to dig trenches, consumers will save time and money, too.

Keep in mind that many wireless units have difficulty transmitting signals through really thick walls or over long distances. Check the specifications on any wireless remote control unit you're considering to make sure it will work in your specific situation.

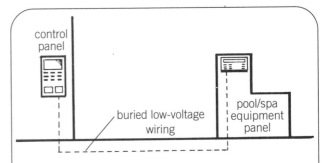

In a hardwired system, information travels via low-voltage wires that connect the control panel to the pool and spa equipment.

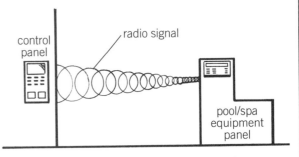

With a radio frequency system, no hardwiring is nec-essary for the control panel to communicate with the pool and spa equipment.

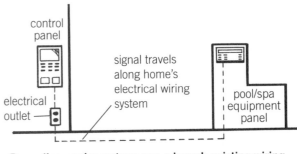

Power line carrier systems use a home's existing wiring to transmit signals to and from the control panel and pool and spa equipment.

POWER LINE CARRIER SYSTEMS

Power line carrier (PLC) systems are more common in general home automa-tion than they are in pool and spa automation. These systems use a home's existing 110-volt electrical wiring to transmit signals from a control center to individual lights and appliances. Basically, a transmitter sends a coded low-voltage digital signal over the home's electrical wiring system. Any PLC receiver plugged into or hardwired to one of the home's outlets will pick up the signal. However, receivers are programmed to respond only to messages sent with a specific address.

Some PLC systems for pools and spas also include wireless remote control for easy poolside monitoring. And like other automation systems, some PLC units incorporate a telephone interface that allows certain functions to be controlled with a simple phone call.

GROWING PAINS

Despite the tremendous advances we've seen in pool and spa automation, many pool builders still haven't fully embraced the new technology, and few pools are being built with these automated features. It's a real shame. After all, you wouldn't think of making a television without a remote control, yet every day pools and spas are being built without automation.

One problem has been that pool builders have been reluctant to learn about the new technology and sell its benefits. Why? Because the controls are perceived as a high-tech installation that many pool builders are unfamiliar with and uncomfortable undertaking.

Also, the pool and spa market is very price sensitive, so builders don't like to introduce anything into the sale that may cause sticker shock — which is possible when you add a $1,000 to $5,000 hardwired automation system to the project. If you've done any shopping for a pool, you may have noticed that many builders start with a base price that includes the necessary equipment and then list the available options, with automation usually at the bottom of the list. That means your pool dealer may never mention automation, and it may be up to you to broach the subject if it's something you think you might want.

Nowadays, savvy consumers — many of whom experience automation technology in their jobs — are embracing automation for the home and demanding it from their pool and spa builders. As consumer demand increases, more and more dealers will be less shy about mentioning it during the sales process.

Another hindrance to pool and spa automation, however, is the lack of standardized protocol between pool and spa manufacturers and the home automation industry. Home automation and pool automation remain hopelessly unintegrated. The home automation industry doesn't know what the pool industry wants or needs, and vice versa. As a result, no one in the market today is handling the automation of the entire home and backyard as one unit.

INDUSTRY LEADERS

Looking for the latest in pool and spa automation systems? Here's a short list of manufacturers leading the charge:

Balboa Instruments
1382 Bell Avenue
Tustin, CA 92780
Phone: 714-384-0384
Web: www.balboa-instruments.com

Innovative Pool Products LLC
1230 North Grove Street, Suite D
Anaheim, CA 92806
Phone: 714-237-1199
Web: www.innovativepools.com

Compool (Pentair Pool Products Inc.)
1620 Hawkins Avenue
Sanford, NC 27330
Phone: 919-774-4151
Web: www.pentairpool.com

Jandy (Waterpik Technologies Inc.)
P.O. Box 6000
Petaluma, CA 94955-6000
Phone: 707-776-8200
Web: www.jandy.com

Hayward Pool Products
620 Division Street
Elizabeth, NJ 07207
Phone: 908-351-5400
Web: www.haywardnet.com

Pentair Pool Products
1620 Hawkins Avenue
Sanford, NC 27330
Phone: 919-774-4151
Web: www.pentairpool.com

Ideally, at the time of new home construction, the home contractor would coordinate with the pool contractor and make sure that the pool automation system could seamlessly integrate with the home automation system. For example, if the new homeowner is soaking in the backyard spa and the glare from the lights inside the home is bothersome, he or she should be able to turn off the house lights from a spa-side control panel. Similarly, a homeowner should be able to control the landscape lights, CD player, and outdoor speakers from the same unit that controls the pool temperature.

Integrating the home and pool/spa automation is paramount if the homeowner is ever going to have a truly leisurely backyard living experience. Clearly, homeowners are not going to want a battalion of control panels on their wall, each one controlling different features of the home. This aspect of home building, however, is undergoing rapid change due to technological advances. Thus, it's easy to envision the day when a single panel controls the entire home and the pool and spa.

In the meantime, some pool and spa automation systems can be adapted to existing home systems. For example, Waterpik Technologies offers adapters that enable its Jandy AquaLink system to "talk" with common communication systems. The AquaLink adapters can plug into any existing control system that has available ports. Then, from the home automation system screen, users can view pool and spa equipment status, turn on or off any device connected to the AquaLink RS unit, view air and water temperatures, and view and/or change pool and spa thermostat settings.

Given how swiftly automation technology has advanced over the past five years, observers believe it won't be long before the sanitation aspect of pools and spas can be as automated as the equipment operation already is. If you're like most homeowners, you have better things to think about than keeping track of your pool and spa. That's where an intelligent control system becomes valuable. It's an investment that really pays off.

Intelligent Control Systems

CONTROL SYSTEM	MANUFACTURER	FUNCTIONS
Aqualink RS OneTouch Control System	Jandy	Allows you to create a custom backyard environment by pressing just one button. As small as a double light switch, the panel controls up to 32 features of the pool, spa, and other backyard amenities.
Wireless AquaLink RS	Jandy	Uses 2.4 GHz radio frequency to control the pool and spa from up to 300 feet away. The wireless technology reduces installation costs (no trenches to dig or conduit to lay), and the system comes with a mountable wall panel or portable desktop model.
CP3800	Compool	Features an electronic timer for spa circulation, pool circulation, and seven auxiliary circuits. It also includes digital thermostats and a temperature display for the pool and spa, a heater cool-down cycle, spa-side remote capability, and automatic freeze protection. The system can be controlled via telephone.
Hayward Pool System Controls	Hayward Pool Products	Offers one-touch programming and easy access to all pool and spa functions. An optional wireless spa-side remote is available, and an integrated dimmer system provides several lighting levels to create the perfect atmosphere.
Simple remote control	Pentair Pool Products	Puts basic pool and spa operation in the palm of your hand.
CP3800	Pentair Pool Products	Puts control of all pool and spa functions at your fingertips.

Pool Amenities

pool or spa environment can be as simple or as elaborate as you want. However, you'll find that you'll enjoy your waterscape even more if you incorporate some ancillary products and amenities — anything from diving boards and slides to fiber-optic lighting and water features. Whereas previous chapters discussed the "must-have" components of a swimming pool or spa, this chapter explores the numerous accessories that turn a ho-hum swimming pool into an aquatic wonderland.

POOL DECKS

For decades, poured concrete has been the material of choice for decking. But many pool owners are turning toward the more upscale look of brick and stone. Like concrete, these materials are durable, but their cost can make them prohibitive for the average consumer — depending on how expansive the deck is. Fortunately, stamped and colored concrete is filling the void between inexpensive poured concrete and pricey stone materials. Stamped-concrete systems enable you to create brick and stone patterns in myriad color schemes to achieve just the look you're seeking. For a truly seamless installation that looks as good as the real thing, hire someone who's experienced with this type of decking material; check out some of his or her installations to get a good sense of his or her work before signing the contract.

Another popular decking choice — especially for spas and aboveground pools — is wood. Decking wood should be a variety that holds up well in wet conditions, such as redwood or cedar. Use only top-grade lumber that's free of imperfections — especially for the deck boards — and make sure the boards are sanded perfectly smooth to eliminate the risk of slivers in bare feet.

For in-ground pools, *wet decks* are a growing trend. Wet decks are recessed an inch or so below the water level of the pool so that water covers them, creating a shallow but wet surface for poolside lounging. Some people install furniture on their wet decks for a cool conversation area, while others use them as a refreshing ledge upon which to sunbathe.

DIVING BOARDS AND JUMPING ROCKS

Diving boards are not as popular as they once were for residential pools because they can easily result in injuries if not installed or used properly. In fact, many builders are wary of liability lawsuits and won't install diving boards on the pools they build. Also, the debate within the industry about what constitutes a safe diving depth in a residential pool continues to this day. The National Spa and Pool Institute and the American National Standards Institute have published standards for builders to follow, but following these standards is no guarantee that an accident won't occur. Given the right physical characteristics of the diver and the right diving projection and velocity, it is still possible for someone to hit the pool bottom or transition wall when diving, possibly resulting in paralysis or death. Thus, utmost care should be taken when installing a diving board, and every user should be trained in proper diving techniques.

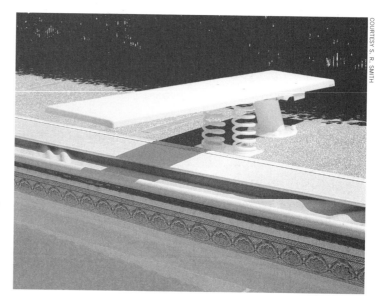

Diving boards are still a popular amenity for residential pools. Before adding a board to your pool, however, make sure that it meets all building standards for diving safety.

Though a diving well will add significant cost to your in-ground pool, the safe enjoyment of a diving board can provide an unparalleled return on your investment.

A jumping rock might be a suitable alternative to a diving board, especially if you have a natural pondlike pool design and don't want to ruin the aesthetic with a diving board. These rocks are usually anchored to the pool structure and seamlessly blend with the rest of the pool coping. They should have a flat, nonslip surface, and the jumping well should be suitable for diving in case some users misuse the rock and dive from it instead of jumping.

SLIDES

Inspired by thrilling waterpark slides, manufacturers of residential swimming pool slides have crafted some exhilarating examples of aquatic flumes. The traditional slide is made of reinforced fiberglass, though some slides are now being made of rotary-molded polyethylene — the same virtually indestructible material used to manufacture much of today's playground equipment. And they are now available in a variety of exciting colors. Because slide material is naturally slippery, water jets are optional. (Though who can resist the lively spray and steady flow of water as it streams down the slide and into the pool below?)

Some slides are designed with modular pieces so you can devise hundreds of configurations, from spirals that take bathers through a dramatic 720-degree twist to embankment slides that wind their way down lengthy hillsides and around trees. Most manufacturers offer slides in several colors, and several offer faux granite designs that blend well with natural or artificial rockwork. Several companies actually encase their slides in faux rock structures that help them blend with today's popular lagoon and rock design pools. Some of these rock encasings even include a water feature on the side, giving you two amenities in one product.

Manufacturers of more traditional pool slides also have hopped on the fashion bandwagon, making available a pleasing palette of colors that enable pool owners to better match slides to home exteriors, tinted concrete decks, and outdoor furniture.

Along with the variety of full-size slides on the market are several kiddie versions. It may seem extravagant to have a slide that no one but the littlest swimmers can use, but it's a whole lot safer than having the kids drag the Little Tikes slide to the pool.

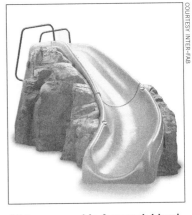

Slides encased in faux rock blend seamlessly with natural pool designs.

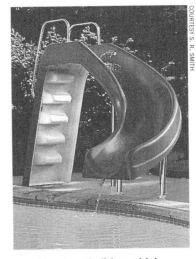

Traditional pool slides, which curve to the left and right, remain popular for families with young children.

All in all, whether you have limited deck space, young children, unique design considerations, or a craving for extreme sports, rest assured there's a pool slide to meet your needs.

WATER FEATURES

As a pool and spa owner, you'll spend more time looking at your aquatic landscape than you'll spend swimming or soaking in it. That's why water features have become one of the most requested pool amenities today. A few popular varieties include:

- **Sheeting waterfalls,** which use a special fitting to produce a curtain of water up to several feet wide. They add drama on raised walls and can be placed over grottoes to create an aquatic doorway.
- **Floating fountains,** which typically hook up to one of the return lines and add interest to an otherwise stagnant pool or spa.
- **Bubbler jets,** which are often used in water features adjacent to a pool. If the water feature is raised above deck level, consider having it spill into the pool for a multidimensional effect.
- **Fountain jets,** which can be mounted under the pool coping to create an arc of water that leaps into the pool. Multiple jets can be timed and choreographed to create an aquatic dance.
- **Misters,** which are popular in arid climates to help cool the ambient temperature. They can create a mystical illusion when incorporated into lush landscapes and surrounding rockwork.

SWIM JETS

If you don't have the space or desire for a lap pool but you want the health benefits of swimming, consider having a swim jet installed at the deep end of your pool. These systems create a continuous current (like a river) that you can swim against. The speed can be dialed up or down for various levels of exercise.

SWIM-OUTS

Swim-outs are underwater benches built into the pool wall, offering a cool respite for those not wanting to venture entirely into the pool. Swim-outs can be fitted with jets to provide cool hydrotherapy. Some people like to install special receptacles for umbrella poles in the pool deck by their swim-outs, allowing loungers in the swim-outs to enjoy some shade.

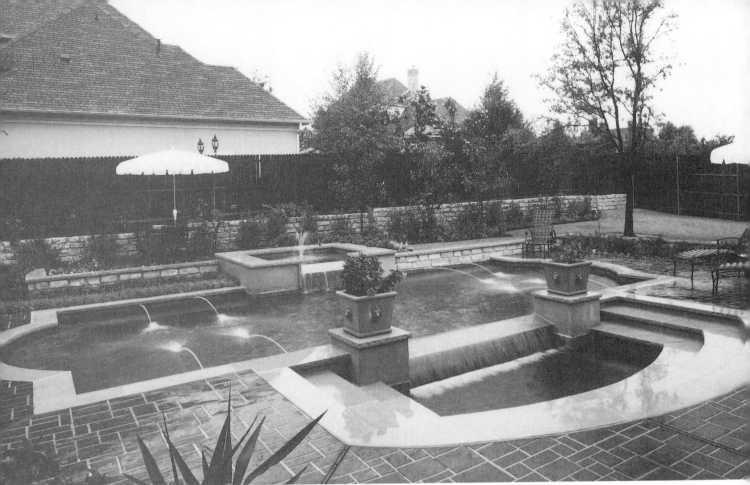

Water features put on a dramatic show at this elaborate pool and spa, which includes eight jets mounted under the coping, a tiered fountain, and two spillways.

FIBER-OPTIC LIGHTING

Eschewing the traditional underwater lights that illuminate a pool at night, an increasing number of pool owners are choosing fiber-optic lighting, which uses fiber-optic cable and a remote illuminator for a wide range of landscape and underwater lighting needs. One of the most popular applications is perimeter lighting, wherein fiber-optic cable is run around the pool's coping to outline the pool with light. Also, many fiber-optic illuminators can be fitted with a color wheel, which enables the user to change the color of the light — from hot red to cool blue, lush green, or clear white — to complement a particular mood.

OUTDOOR/UNDERWATER SPEAKERS

For the music lover, outdoor speakers are a must for creating a resort atmosphere in your own backyard. And if you never want to miss a beat, consider extending the sound to your pool with underwater speakers. These are best installed by a professional at the time the pool is built.

CASUAL FURNITURE

It's impossible to enjoy your pool or spa setting without the use of outdoor furniture. But before you buy, make sure the furniture is suitable for a pool or spa environment.

- ~ Lightweight PVC furniture can blow into your in-ground pool or spa and damage the surface, especially with vinyl-lined pools.
- ~ Wood furniture should be able to withstand lots of moisture from wet bathers and towels. A good choice would be teak, redwood, or some other weather-resistant variety.
- ~ If you plan to use cushions or fabric, make sure they're designed for outdoor use. Outdoor fabrics are formulated to resist fading, mold, and mildew. Some fabrics, however, may not hold up well if constantly exposed to chlorinated pool water.
- ~ Choose a seating material that will dry quickly, so that those who don't want to get wet can lounge poolside without the concern that a wet bather may have just used the furniture. Most non-cushioned, non-fabric designs dry quickly.
- ~ Have adequate seating where you want it. This may require investing in multiple furniture groupings so you have the seating conveniently located for dining, poolside conversation, breaks from the hot tub, and so on.

TOYS AND GAMES

Sure, Marco Polo is a fun water game, but investing in the right toys and games will ensure that you never get bored with your pool purchase. Toys and games are a must for any pool owner with children, or for anyone with a child-like enthusiasm for swimming. From simple beach balls and inflatable rafts to water noodles and diving rings, toys add countless hours of enjoyment to the pool experience. In fact, many of today's pools are designed for recreation, starting at the ends with a depth of 3 feet (0.9 m) and sloping to a center depth of 5 feet (1.5 m). The center slope makes a pool ideally suited for water volleyball, basketball, or any number of games. If you're a big volleyball fan, you may want to have sockets for the net poles set right into the deck for easy set-up and tear-down. For basketball fans, there are numerous poolside hoops available on the market.

Make sure that any toys you buy are appropriate and safe for the age of the children who will be playing with them. And never rely on inflatable toys to safeguard poor swimmers.

OUTDOOR KITCHENS

One of the biggest trends in poolscape design is the use of outdoor kitchens to focus all the family and entertaining activities around the pool. These al fresco kitchens can include not only built-in barbecue grills but also running water, refrigerators, and even wood-fired ovens.

OUTDOOR FIREPLACES AND HEATERS

Whether wood-burning or fueled by natural gas, outdoor fireplaces are all the rage for creating nighttime ambience and taking the chill out of the air. For greater flexibility on where the heat goes, you may want to consider purchasing a couple of outdoor heaters, which use LP gas tanks. Tabletop or floor models allow you to place the heat where you need it most. Either way, outdoor fireplaces and heaters make it possible to enjoy your outdoor pool and spa even when the weather suggests otherwise.

POOL HOUSES AND GAZEBOS

If you're a pool owner who embraces the outdoor living concept, a pool house probably is on your wish list. Once built to house the pool equipment and changing facilities, modern pool houses now double as guest homes, with fully equipped kitchens, bathrooms, and comfortable rooms for relaxation out of the sun. Often a pool house is the best way to keep heavy traffic out of the main residence during pool parties or even on normal summer days when the kids are in and out of the pool all day long.

For spas, many people opt for a gazebo, which creates privacy and offers protection from the elements. Some gazebos are just large enough to house the spa, while others are big enough for small social gatherings.

Winterizing a Pool or Spa

One of the saddest days of the year is the day you decide it's time to put your pool or spa to sleep for the winter. Of course, if you live in the Sun Belt or some other region where the weather permits year-round swimming, there's no need to shut down your pool. And many spa owners find wintry soaks in the hot tub to be an exhilarating adventure that's well worth the cost of heating the tub throughout the snowy season.

For those of you, however, who must shut down your pool or spa for the winter, keep reading. This chapter takes you step-by-step through the winterizing process.

WINTERIZING A POOL

Mid-September is the traditional time for pool closings. The days are getting shorter, the weather is getting colder, and the leaves are about to fall and make a mess at the bottom of your pool. Though it's not something most pool owners like to think about, closing the pool is one of the most important tasks you'll have as a pool owner. It's much easier to reopen a pool in the springtime if it's been properly winterized the previous fall. So all the hard work you put into it in September will save you countless hours next May when you're anxious to get things up and running again.

All pools differ somewhat, which may mean you'll have some special closing procedures to follow. If after reading this chapter you still have concerns about how to close your pool, contact your trusty pool professional. Meanwhile, the following general guidelines are sufficient for most pool owners.

1. Assemble All Your Winterizing Supplies and Equipment

Gather all of your supplies before you get started. These include your winterizing chemicals, plugs for the skimmers and return jets, the pool cover (if it's in storage), and an air compressor or shop vac. If your cover is an automatic or manual reel cover, you're all set.

2. Balance and Shock the Water

Check the pH and get it as close to 7.4 as possible. Then super-chlorinate (shock) the water with unstabilized chlorine to kill any algae that may be present and to help maintain water clarity during the winter months. It's a good idea to add a winter algaecide and a stain preventive at this time. Many pool supply stores sell winterizing kits that package all these chemicals together for your convenience.

If possible, balance and shock the water the day before you intend to put the pool to bed to allow the water to circulate and mix up the chemicals.

> **CAUTION!**
> Never leave chlorine tablets or floating chemical dispensers in the pool over the winter, because the water won't be circulating and the concentration of chemicals in one area can cause damage, especially to vinyl-lined pools.

3. Clean the Filters

Clean cartridge filters and backwash sand and DE filters as you normally would. For sand and DE filters, leave the backwash valve open. Don't acid-wash DE filters at this time, even if you plan to rinse off the acid with clean water. Acid residue could remain on the filter grid and damage the filter during the winter months. You can acid-wash the filter grids in the spring, if necessary, when you can immediately run pool water through the system.

4. Disconnect the Electricity and Gas

Before working on the electrical equipment, turn off the power at the breaker box. If you have a gas heater, turn off the gas supply. You may want to tape over these switches to prevent someone from accidentally turning them on during the winter months.

5. Drain and Disconnect the Filter

No matter which type of filter you have, drain it and leave the drain plug off. A good place to store the drain plug is in the pump basket; then you can locate it easily in the spring. To ensure that no water remains in the filter's multi-port valve, blow air through it with a compressor or suck water out of it with a shop vac. Unless you have a sand filter, which would be too heavy to move, consider storing your filter in a garage or storage shed to protect it from the elements.

6. Drain and Disconnect the Pump

Make sure there is no water in the pump. Remove any drain plugs and store them in the pump basket. Turn the pump upside down to make sure all the water has run out. Even a little trapped water can cause damage when it freezes. Store the pump in a garage or storage shed.

7. Drain and Disconnect the Heater

If you have a heater, you may have been able to postpone closing your pool for a few weeks. But eventually the time comes when even heated pools need to be winterized. As with the other pieces of equipment, the heater must be drained. Force all the water out with either a compressor or a shop vac. (You've turned off the electricity and gas beforehand, right?) Remove the heater tray only if recommended by the manufacturer.

For solar heaters, drain all water from the solar panels.

8. Disconnect All Unions and Remove All Return Jets

Even a little water trapped in a fitting can cause a freeze crack to occur, so make sure all water is drained from the circulation system by disconnecting all fittings and unions. Also remove return jet fittings.

HIRING PROFESSIONALS

Considering the financial investment you've made in your pool, you might want to let a reputable pool service company or your pool builder winterize the pool, at least for the first winter after it's installed. You can then observe the procedure and do it yourself the next year, if you want. A reputable company will stand behind its winterizing work. That's important, because if winterizing is not correctly done in a cold climate, it can result in thousands of dollars of repair work the following spring. If you do hire a service company, read the service contract carefully and ask questions. Most companies will not assume responsibility for staining over the winter months or damage caused by unusual weather conditions.

9. Remove Water from the Return Lines

Use an air compressor or a shop vac to remove water from all return lines. You can hook up an air compressor or shop vac to the return lines at the filter system. Keep the air blowing until bubbles are flowing full force from the return jets in the pool. Working underwater, put a plug in each fitting and make sure it's tight.

10. Remove Water from the Suction Lines

Use an air compressor or a shop vac to remove water from all suction lines. You can hook up an air compressor or shop vac to the suction lines at the skimmer. When air is flowing full force from the skimmer, screw a Gizzmo-style device into the skimmer. A Gizzmo is the brand name for a device that absorbs the pressure of freezing water so that the forming ice doesn't damage the skimmer. You can purchase these from pool supply stores. Some Gizzmo-like devices require that you put Teflon tape on the threads to guarantee a tight seal.

There are other items you can use to absorb the expansion of water as it freezes in the skimmer. Even a capped plastic soda bottle will work. Whatever you do, however, don't leave the skimmer without anything to absorb the pressure of the ice. Otherwise, the skimmer will likely crack.

For aboveground pools, you have the option of removing the skimmer completely and installing a winter plate over the hole in the pool wall. You may also opt to lower the water level below the skimmer line.

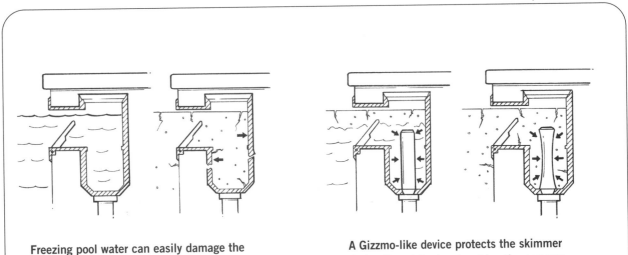

Freezing pool water can easily damage the skimmer.

A Gizzmo-like device protects the skimmer during the winter by absorbing the pressure caused by freezing water.

ANTIFREEZE

There is no need to add antifreeze to your pool's plumbing system if you properly remove all the water from the lines. Antifreeze is difficult to clean up in the spring and will find its way into your swimming pool water. If you can't remove the water from the pipes for some reason, use only antifreeze recommended for swimming pools. Never use automobile antifreeze.

11. Drain Water from All Accessories

Use an air compressor or a shop vac to remove water from all other amenities and accessories connected to the circulation system, such as waterslides, waterfalls, and automatic cleaning systems. For aboveground pools, remove ladders, slides, and grab rails.

12. Remove Water from the Main Drain

If your pool has a main drain, blow the water out and plug the pipe at the equipment end. This creates an airlock and prevents water from reentering the main drain.

13. Close All Exposed Pipe Ends

Use tape (duct tape works well) to close all exposed pipes to prevent water and debris from entering the circulation system.

14. Adjust the Water Level

There is some controversy when it comes to the proper water level for a winterized pool. Some experts recommend draining the pool below the skimmer, but this isn't necessary if you've successfully removed all the water from the plumbing lines and properly plugged the skimmer and pipes as outlined above. The main exception is if you have a pool with ceramic tile along the waterline; in this case, you may want to drop the water level below the tile so that pressure from the expanding ice doesn't crack the tile.

There are some advantages to keeping the water level high. A high water level helps support the pool cover so that it doesn't sag excessively and become stressed. Also, in areas with high water tables, it's important to keep the pool's water level high so that pressure from groundwater doesn't damage the pool structure or force the pool shell to pop out of the ground. After all, an empty pool shell is not unlike a boat, which prefers to float atop the water. Keeping the water level in the pool high will keep the shell from rising above the groundwater. In addition, if you keep the pool's water level high, you don't have to remove any underwater pool lights because they'll remain below the freezing point.

15. Install the Pool Cover

Make sure your cover is in good condition and repair any cuts or tears as needed. Install the cover according to the manufacturer's instructions.

For aboveground pools, air pillows are often used to absorb the pressure of expanding ice. These can be purchased from pool supply stores. If you can't find one, you can also use inner tubes, beach balls, or other inflatable items. Attach these items at two or more points around the pool to keep them anchored toward the center of the pool.

If water collects on the surface of the cover, be sure to remove it promptly with a shop vac or small pump. Standing water — even the slightest amount — presents a safety hazard.

OFF-SEASON CARE

In milder climates, where there is little risk of freezing, pool care is simply a continuation of normal seasonal pool care, but there is less of it. With swimming at a minimum, there is not as much need for chemical sanitizing and filtration. Colder temperatures and reduced swimming greatly cut down on the growth of algae or bacteria. You may have some problem with leaves in the fall, but regular use of a pool cover alleviates this problem.

Though the weather may be too cool for regular swimming, many pool owners still enjoy the sights and sounds their pools offer. Waterfalls, for example, are still dramatic to look at even if they cascade into water that's too cold to swim in.

When the daytime temperatures are too cold for swimming, it's time to turn off the pool heater if you have one. Some experts recommend that the pilot light be left on to prevent moisture from collecting in the lines. With the heater off, you'll want to pay attention to any severe drops in temperature. If the forecast calls for near-freezing temperatures, set the circulation system to run nonstop. If you have a heater, you'll want to turn it back on to its lowest setting.

When there is no threat of freezing temperatures, the pool's filtering cycle can usually be cut in half.

During the winter months, you'll still check water balance (pH, calcium hardness, and chlorine residual) once a week and adjust to appropriate levels. Also check and clean out the skimmer box and pump leaf strainer faithfully. If the pool is uncovered, you should still vacuum and brush the walls when they begin to look dirty. This will reduce the chances of staining.

Wherever you live, the routine or preparation for the winter months is an essential part of proper pool maintenance. Treat your pool well during this crucial season and it will reward you with many years of trouble-free fun and excitement.

WINTERIZING SPAS

There's no reason not to use your hot tub during the winter months. Even if you don't feel like braving snowdrifts and icicles in your bathrobe to enjoy a steamy soak beneath the wintry sky, you can still leave your spa running for just pennies a day to ensure that the water doesn't freeze and damage the equipment and plumbing.

Yet if your spa is located at a summer vacation home that you're not likely to visit for several months, you may want to winterize the spa just in case the power goes out during a winter storm and you're not there to attend to the spa before it freezes up.

If you choose to shut down your spa for the winter, be careful. Even a little water in the lines or equipment can cause extensive damage that's costly to repair. With that said, here are some general steps you should follow when winterizing your hot tub.

1. Disconnect the Electricity

Switch off the spa at the circuit breaker and trip the ground fault circuit interrupter (GFCI). If the spa isn't hardwired, unplug it from its outlet.

2. Drain the Spa

Drain the spa by hooking up a garden hose to the spa's drain spout. You shouldn't need to create a siphon as long as the spa's drain is above the discharge end of the hose. You can also force the water with a small submersible pump. In either case, leave the drain spout open so that water can't accumulate there and freeze.

If your spa is gunite and has air jets or an air channel under the spa seats, you'll need to blow the air out of the system. To do this, turn off or disconnect the spa heater and pumps and then switch the circuit breaker back on. (Turning off the heater and pumps ensures that the equipment doesn't accidentally overheat in the absence of circulating water.) Activate the spa's air blower and let it run for about 30 seconds. This will blow all the water out of the air channel. This step is not necessary for prefabricated acrylic spas.

Soak up all of the remaining water from inside the spa with a towel, sponge, or mop, or suck it out with a shop vac. Make sure that you get out all the water, especially in the foot well. Some experts recommend leaving a large absorbent towel in the foot well to soak up water that might settle there.

Remove the cartridge filter from the spa and make sure that all the water is out of the filter canister compartment. Store the cartridge in the garage or some other dry place where it won't be exposed to harsh weather conditions.

3. Remove All Fittings and Drain Plugs

Unscrew or disconnect any fittings on your spa equipment that look like they could be taken apart. These are usually located on either side of the heater and the pump. Removing the fittings allows any trapped water to flow out. Also remove any drain plugs that may be on the pump housing, filter canister, or heater to prevent any freezing water from cracking the casings.

4. Remove Water from the Jets

With the topside air controls closed, use a shop vac or compressor to blow out any water standing in the jet plumbing. Get into the spa and put the blowing end of the hose up against each jet. Start with the jet closest to the return side of the pump and work your way around the spa. As you do this, more water will pour out of the various fittings you unscrewed on the equipment. This will remove most of the water from your spa system and greatly reduce the chance of water freezing and causing damage. Don't put any antifreeze in your spa or equipment. Rather, make sure you've done the above steps properly to remove all the water.

5. Install the Cover and Any Panels

Secure the hard cover to the spa with latching straps or other devices so that it can't be dislodged by strong winds. On portable spas with cabinets, replace and secure all panels you may have removed to access the equipment compartment.

Some people secure a tarp over their spa cover and cabinet to further protect them from the harsh winter elements. This can also be a good idea for in-ground or in-deck spas to prevent rainwater from entering the spa.

Opening a Pool or Spa

he best way to ensure that opening your pool in the spring is a cinch is to make sure you close it properly the previous fall. If you don't, you could encounter a dirty, algae-laden pool; frost-damaged equipment and pipes; cracked tiles; damaged vinyl liners; and a host of other problems. The procedures for closing pools and spas are covered in the previous chapter. If you heed that advice, your spring cleanup will be a breeze. Just follow the basic steps in this chapter, and you'll be ready to swim or soak in as little as one day.

OPENING A POOL

As with winterizing a pool, you may opt to have a service company open your pool for you. In fact, if you hired a company to winterize your pool, it might be best to have the same company reopen your pool because its service technicians will be familiar with any unique situations your pool presents. However, if you successfully winterized the pool yourself, you should be able to open it yourself with little difficulty. Here's how.

1. Clean the Cover and Deck

Before you even think about removing the cover, clean the deck area to prevent any debris from being swept into the pool. This will also give you a nice working area for cleaning and preparing the cover for storage. Use a pump to remove any standing water on the cover. Then use a hose and broom to clear away any dirt and debris from the cover. Now if the cover slips into the pool while you're removing it, you won't be dumping a lot of debris and dirty water into the pool.

2. Remove and Store the Cover

Carefully remove the cover and lay it out on the deck. Depending on the size of your pool and the type of cover you have, this may require a few people. Clean the cover according to the manufacturer's instructions (usually with a stiff brush and mild detergent), then allow it to dry thoroughly before folding it up for storage. After the cover has been cleaned, dried, and folded, store it in a clean, dry place away from the sun.

If your cover needs water tubes to secure it in place, you should empty them now and clean them for storage. For aboveground pools, remove the air pillow, deflate it, and store it.

3. Remove the Plugs

If the pool was winterized properly, there should be plugs in all the fittings where equipment and hoses were attached to the pool. The plugs kept water out of the cleared lines so that it couldn't freeze and crack the pipes. Remove them now.

If your pool was winterized with antifreeze, you'll need to lower the water level until it's below the blocked lines. Then remove the plugs — one at a time — and drain the antifreeze into a bucket. You may need to use a compressor or shop vac to clear the lines of antifreeze.

4. Reconnect the Light Fixtures

In some regions, pool companies insist on lowering the pool water level when winterizing. This means that the light fixtures need to be removed because they could crack when the water freezes. If the pool is not drained, the light fixtures can be left alone because the water shouldn't freeze at that depth. If your light fixtures were removed from their wall niches, now's the time to replace them.

5. Reconnect Deck Equipment

Sometimes when a pool is winterized, deck equipment — such as ladders, handrails, diving boards, and slides — are removed and stored. Now's the time to reattach them. Make sure you reconnect any grounding wires that were attached to metal parts. It's a good idea to lubricate all bolts on the diving board, ladders, and rails to prevent them from rusting during the summer. This will make them much easier to remove next fall.

6. Reinstall the Skimmer Baskets and Fittings

For aboveground pools, the entire skimmer may have been removed and a winter plate installed in its place. Replace the skimmer now. Also hook up any hoses from the skimmer and return jets that lead to the pump and filter.

For all pools, insert the skimmer basket and reinstall the return jet fittings that were removed when the pool was winterized.

7. Examine the Pool Shell

If you have a concrete or fiberglass pool, look for cracks or surface irregularities in the shell. If you have a vinyl-lined pool, look for tears and washouts. A washout occurs when excessive groundwater (due to heavy rains or quick thaws) erodes the sand beneath the pool's vinyl floor, which may result in the liner resting on sharp rocks and stones. Also look at the pool coping and waterline tile to make sure it's in good condition.

Repairs should be made now, before you open the pool for swimming. Most shell repairs should be addressed by a pool professional. Some minor repairs, such as a small tear in a vinyl liner — can be done yourself with a kit available from pool supply stores. (See chapter 16 for more information.)

If you do need to call in a professional, don't wait another minute. Spring is an extremely busy time for pool professionals, who may be out in the field opening pools for hundreds of homeowners. The longer you wait to call, the farther down on the waiting list your job goes.

8. Clean the Tile

Clean any scale or stains from the tile so that it looks as good as new.

9. Reconnect the Pump, Filter, and Heater

If no repairs need to be made to the pool structure, or once they have been made, it's time to reinstall the pump (if you removed it), the filter, and the heater (if you have one). Check and reconnect the wiring and pipes. Make sure all the fittings are clean and tight, and replace any drainage plugs, valves, and pressure gauges that were removed for the winter. If you have booster pumps for water features or an automatic pool cleaner, reinstall them, too.

Check the filter for cracks in its casing. If you have a sand filter, remove any mud balls that have formed. If you have a DE filter, get prepared to add a slurry of diatomaceous earth and water to it, according to the manufacturer's guidelines.

Make sure any grounding wires are properly connected to equipment that needs them.

10. Fill the Pool

Make sure the water level is at the proper height.

11. Turn On the Power

When the pool was winterized, the power should have been turned off at the circuit breaker. Now you can switch it back on, leaving the equipment turned off until you can get back to the pool. Set all equipment timers and switches to their normal operating position.

12. Check Valves and Fill the Pump

Make sure that all valves are in the open position, but bypass the filter for now until you're sure the system is flowing properly. Fill the pump with water to make sure it primes properly. You can do this by pouring water in through the leaf trap. Make sure the skimmer weir (or flap) is operating correctly.

13. Start Up the Pool System

Make sure the pump primes and the system flows properly. Look for leaks, split hoses, and cracks throughout the system. When you first start the filtration system after a long period of disuse, you may notice that some valves are leaking. The leaks could be the result of dried-out gaskets; once the gaskets are wet, the leaks may stop. If the valves don't stop leaking, they probably require new gaskets or may have a structural defect, in which case they will have to be replaced. Turn off the power until a service technician has made the necessary repairs.

14. Backwash the Filter

To prevent previously trapped debris from entering the pool, backwash sand and DE filters thoroughly. Be prepared to add a fresh slurry of diatomaceous earth and water to your DE filter when you switch back to normal filtration. If you're using a cartridge filter, make sure the cartridge is clean in case you didn't clean it thoroughly when you winterized. If you're having any trouble with the filter, check out chapter 7 or consult with a pool professional.

15. Treat the Water

If the pool is relatively clear, test for sanitizer residual, pH, and alkalinity. Make sure you are using fresh test strips and/or reagents in your test kit to ensure proper readings. Add the appropriate chemicals to bring these water-balance factors into their proper ranges (see chapter 4 for more information). Most professionals recommend shocking the pool water upon reopening the pool to kill any bacteria and algae and to burn up any organic waste in the water. Shocks are available in liquid and granular form, and you'll want to add enough to raise the chlorine level to 3.0 ppm (parts per million). Mix and apply the chemicals according to the directions on the packaging to avoid damage to the pool surface and equipment.

If your pool is green with algae, the shock will help, but you may also need to add an algaecide.

It's important that you test, balance, and treat the water as soon as possible. After the pool cover is removed, sunlight will greatly accelerate the growth of algae and bacteria, making them harder to treat.

16. Run the Filtration System until the Pool Is Clean

After letting the filter run for 24 hours, vacuum any debris from the bottom and retest the water. Don't let anyone swim in the pool until the water is properly balanced and sanitized. It may take several days of filter operation to clarify a pool. Some experts recommend reducing the pump operation one hour per day until you reach your normal filtration cycle time. During the first few days of operation, you may need to backwash or clean the filter several times, depending on how dirty the water was when you started.

OPENING A SPA

Opening a spa or hot tub after a winter hiatus is simply a matter of reversing the steps taken to winterize the spa. If the spa was winterized properly, there's little that can go wrong. If the spa wasn't winterized properly, then much is at risk.

Assuming your spa was winterized properly (see chapter 13), follow the basic steps outlined below to reopen it. Your spa may have some unique issues that your spa professional will have to help you with. These guidelines, however, are sufficient for the vast majority of residential spas.

1. Remove the Tarp/Cover

If you covered your spa with a tarp for the winter, remove it. Clean the tarp and allow it to dry before storing it. Then remove the spa's insulating cover.

2. Clean the Shell

Drain any water that found its way inside the spa, and clean away any dirt. Inspect the shell for cracks or splits, especially if water got into the spa shell and froze. Any damage to the spa shell should be repaired by a spa professional before going any further.

Once you've wiped out any water or dirt and inspected the shell for damage, use an acrylic cleanser to clean the shell. Don't use any cleaners that contain harsh abrasives that could scratch the shell. Then rinse the cleanser from the surface and drain away the dirty water from the inside of the tub.

Some experts recommend waxing an acrylic spa shell at this point to restore its luster. Use only an acrylic wax, not a variety designed for automobiles or furniture. Use a soft cotton cloth to buff the surface to a shiny finish.

3. Clean the Filter

If you didn't clean the filter when you winterized the spa, clean it now. You may need to use a special cartridge filter cleaner to remove deposits on the filter element. Such specialty cleaners are available from your spa dealer. Then reinstall the filter in the spa.

4. Clean the Cover

Most spa covers are made of a foam core surrounded by vinyl. Over time, the vinyl can dry out and crack. To extend the life of your spa cover, you should clean it and condition it. Follow the instructions on page 121.

5. Reassemble the Spa Equipment

If the spa was winterized properly, a number of fittings for the equipment should have been left unscrewed or open. Make sure these are all reconnected and tightened. Close any drains that were left open. Look around for any obvious signs of winter damage, such as cracks where water may have been overlooked and allowed to freeze. If there's a problem, call in the professionals.

If you have an external gas heater, make sure the gas is properly connected and all heater parts are in good working condition. If you smell gas, turn off the gas and call in the professionals immediately.

6. Fill the Spa

Fill the spa with fresh water and observe it for possible leaks as water flows into all the jet tubing and equipment. If there are any leaks, stop the water and fix them immediately. Leaks at fittings may indicate a need for new gaskets or O-rings.

7. Turn On the Power

Once the spa has been filled, turn on the power. First switch the circuit breaker for the spa back on (it should have been turned off when the spa was winterized), then check the GFCI (ground fault circuit interrupter) for the spa to make sure it works properly.

Check the spa operation. Use the control panel to make sure each pump, air blower, light, and any other spa feature is working properly. If you don't have adequate flow through the heater, you could burn out the elements rather quickly.

8. Balance the Water

Balance the water and adjust the sanitizer level. Wait for the spa to heat up to the desired temperature and retest the water. Make any necessary adjustments. See chapter 4 for more information.

Once the water is balanced, you can slip in and enjoy!

TROUBLESHOOTING

Does this sound familiar? Just when you've gotten excited about getting your pool up and running for another fun-filled summer, some problem pops up. Don't fret. The chart on the facing page is a list of some pool start-up problems and how to deal with them.

Troubleshooting Start-Up

PROBLEM	SOLUTION
Water is dripping from the filter, pump, or plumbing.	Tighten the fittings and inspect hoses for cracks. You may need to replace gaskets in some of your valves if they're worn out. If you can't get the leaks to stop, contact a pool professional.
Sand or DE is settling on the bottom of the pool near the return jets.	A cracked filter component could be sending sand or DE back into the pool. Take the filter apart and make any necessary repairs. You may need to contact a pool professional depending on which part is damaged. There's also a possibility that an underground pipe is leaking, which could allow sand into the pool. If this is the case, you may be losing water as well. Contact a pool professional to make the repair.
Filter output is low.	Backwash your sand or DE filter or clean your cartridge filter, depending on which type you have. If the output is still low, you may have a cracked filter component that's sending sand or DE back into the pool. Also, a DE filter may need its grids acid-washed, and a sand filter may need a change of sand. If that fails, contact a pool professional.
Air bubbles are coming out of the return jets.	This usually means there's a leak somewhere along the suction line, often near the skimmer. If that's the case, it's time to call in the professionals. This is not a repair for the unskilled.
There's a depression in the ground, or patio blocks and stones are sinking.	This could mean that you have a leak in an underground pipe that's washing away soil and causing the depression. This is a repair for the professionals.
The pump makes a screeching noise and/or does not seem to run properly.	After sitting idle all winter, a pump can encounter problems when it's restarted in the spring. Either take the pump in for repair or replace it if you think it's on its last legs anyway.
The pool is losing water.	If you notice the water level in the pool dropping, it may be caused by more than mere evaporation. Chances are the winter's freeze and thaw has caused some structural damage that needs immediate attention. Finding the source of a leak can be like finding the veritable needle in a haystack. In fact, leak detection is a whole industry unto itself, and you may need to call in the pros to locate and patch a leak. Sometimes you can home in on the leak. If the pool water level drops to the bottom of the skimmer and then stops, the leak is probably on the suction side of the pool equipment. If the pool water level goes down to the bottom of the return jets and then stops, this usually means there is a leak somewhere along the return line. Similarly, if the leak goes down to the light niche, the leak is probably related to the light fixture. If the water stops at any other point, the leak may be due to a crack in the pool wall or a tear in the vinyl liner at that point. If the water keeps draining out, you may have a leak in the pool floor — which is the worst possible place. With the exception of a small vinyl-liner repair, all leaks should be repaired by a trained professional.

15 Pool and Spa Safety

Accidental drowning is the leading cause of death for children under the age of 5, and most of these incidents could have been prevented with proper adult supervision. Too often we hear stories of a guardian who turned his or her attention away from the pool for just a moment — maybe to answer the phone or freshen a glass of lemonade — only to discover that in the space of that moment a toddler had drowned.

But young children aren't the only ones at risk around pools and spas. Teenagers who are allowed to horseplay on diving boards and pool decks have been known to suffer head and neck injuries, sometimes resulting in paralysis. Adults — particularly when under the influence of alcohol — have been known to exercise poor judgment and become injured in backyard pools and spas. Adults — especially the elderly — have drowned in hot tubs after soaking for too long in water that's been too hot for their system to handle; when they stand up, they become dizzy and sometimes faint into the water.

Clearly, pools and spas can pose a danger to anyone who misuses them, regardless of age. As a pool and spa owner, you have an inherent responsibility to ensure that your pool and spa environment doesn't pose an unreasonable danger to neighbors or guests and that youngsters' aquatic activities are properly supervised at all times. This chapter reviews the various safety precautions you should take to ensure that you, your family, and your guests have a safe and enjoyable time in your pool and spa.

SAFETY IN NUMBERS

One theory of pool and spa safety says that the more safety products you use around your aquatic environment, the less chance there is that someone will accidentally drown. The idea is that each safety device will act like a checkpoint through which someone must pass before reaching the water. If someone slips by one checkpoint undetected, ideally they'll be stopped at the next checkpoint. Some of these checkpoints could include an automatic safety cover, a fence, and an alarm on the door to the pool.

Multiple checkpoints may help deter uninvited guests from entering your pool and spa area, but they'll never replace the need for adult supervision. After all, fences can be left unlocked, door alarms can be switched off, and automatic pool covers can be left open. Even so, safety products can provide more than peace of mind; they can truly prevent accidents if used according to the manufacturers' instructions.

Here's a brief look at some of the most common safety products you may want to consider as you set up safety checkpoints around your pool and spa.

Fencing

You may not have a choice regarding whether to put up fencing around your pool and spa. Many municipalities require such fencing and dictate the style and design of fencing you must use. A safety fence should be at least 48 inches (122 cm) high and not have any openings a child might squeeze through. It should also be extremely difficult to get a hand- or toehold on the fence for climbing. Fences that are surrounded by thorny shrubs and flower beds are less likely to be climbed than those that offer a clear runway. Also, fences that allow outsiders to see into the pool and spa area are less of a deterrent than those that block the view of the pool and spa entirely.

A few common styles of pool and spa fencing include chain link, ornamental wrought iron or aluminum, and wooden picket. Another option that's increasingly popular is portable fencing, which typically consists of metal poles and durable netting that can be installed around a

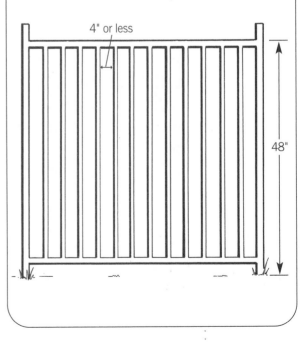

Install the fence completely around the pool. It should be at least 4 feet high and have no footholds or handholds to help a young child climb it. Vertical fence slats should be 4 inches or less apart to keep a child from squeezing through.

4" or less

48"

pool deck when needed and easily dissembled when not needed. Before you decide on a fence style, however, make sure that it meets all of the building code requirements in your area.

Safety Covers

Safety covers provide an impenetrable barrier between the water and the unauthorized visitor.

For spas, the thermal insulating cover can double as the safety cover if it has locking straps that hold it down.

For pools, the best solution is an automatic or manual safety cover that runs on tracks. With automatic units, the cover is powered with a motor that is operated by a key or an electronic control. Manual units must be physically pulled across the pool and retracted with a hand-wrench device. Either style provides superior safety if it's placed over the pool every time the area is left unsupervised.

Another type of pool safety cover is the tie-down variety, which anchors to the deck with special straps and hardware. These work extremely well to safeguard the pool during long periods of nonuse — such as when the pool is winterized — but they are often too cumbersome for day-to-day use.

See chapter 10 for more information on pool and spa covers.

Self-Latching Gates

A self-latching gate has a mechanism that automatically closes the gate and latches it securely. To pass through the gate, a person must be able to undo the latch in order to push or pull the gate open. To prevent unauthorized entry by small children and toddlers, the latch should be placed well above a child's reach and the gate designed to discourage climbing.

Self-Closing Doors

Similar to a self-latching gate, a self-closing door automatically closes and latches itself each time someone passes through. Most doors leading from the home to the pool or spa area can be converted into a self-closing door with the use of special hardware, such as hinge pins, swing arms, and sliding glass door closers. Check with a home improvement store for advice on converting your pool- or spa-side doors into self-closing barriers.

Door Alarms

Door alarms can be installed on all doors leading from the home to the pool or spa area. Typically, these devices sound an alarm when someone passes through without first triggering the "pass" or "reset" button. Door alarms are especially useful when small children are in the house and it's impossible to keep a watchful eye on them at all times. With a door alarm, a baby-sitter or adult supervisor should have ample opportunity to fetch an errant child before he or she has time to get to the pool or spa. Obviously, it's important to keep the reset button out of a child's reach. It's also imperative that adults in the house not disarm the alarm because they're annoyed by having to hit the reset button every time they pass through the door. Like all safety products, door alarms work only if they're used properly and consistently.

Pool Alarms

Pool alarms come in a variety of styles and designs. Some detect wave motion on the surface of the water, while others pick up on motion under the water. A major concern with such pool alarms is that they sound off *after* someone has already entered the water, which may, perhaps, not permit enough time for a rescue effort.

Electronic surveillance systems provide a bit more warning by sounding an alarm after someone has entered a defined area. In recent times, infrared technology has been adapted to pool alarms. These devices surround the pool and spa area with an infrared light beam that's bounced around by mirrors stacked on the ground. When the beam is broken — whether by a child or a pet passing through it — an alarm sounds. The infrared units are designed not to sound a false alarm if leaves or debris blow through the infrared beam.

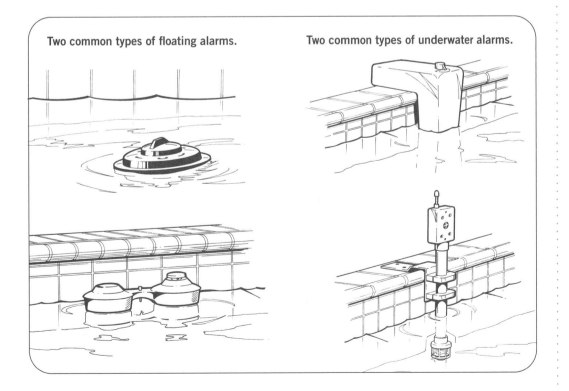

Two common types of floating alarms.

Two common types of underwater alarms.

Sometimes two or more units are needed to surround the pool or spa with an infrared beam.

When shopping for alarms, make sure the alarm is suitable for your situation. Some alarms are so sensitive that heavy winds can cause enough motion on the water surface to trigger the alarm. The U.S. Consumer Product Safety Commission has tested some of the pool alarms on the market. The commission found that "underwater alarms generally performed better than surface alarms." During testing, which simulated the action of a small child falling into the pool, the underwater alarms were more consistent in alarming and less likely to sound false alarms than the other types of alarms. As an added bonus, some underwater alarms can be used in conjunction with pool covers, whereas the surface alarms cannot.

Regardless of the type of alarm you choose, it's important to use remote alarm receivers so the alarm can be heard inside the house.

Personal Alarms

Personal alarms are somewhat new on the pool and spa scene. These devices consist of a base unit and a remote device that attaches to a child. When the remote travels beyond a certain distance from the base unit or when it's submerged in water, it triggers the alarm. These units are sometimes marketed to pet owners, as well, because dogs and cats sometimes fall or jump into a pool and then can't find their way to the steps or a ladder to climb out.

Floating Swimwear

Floating swimwear is essentially a spandex swimsuit with a foam core that helps keep children buoyant. Like water wings, floating swimwear should not be relied on to protect a child from drowning. If you opt to use floating swimwear with your children, make sure that the suits zip up the back so that children can't remove them on their own. Some pool supply stores sell floating swimwear, but you might also be able to find it at your local sporting goods store.

Rescue Equipment

Having the appropriate rescue equipment on hand can mean the difference between life and death. Every pool should be equipped with the basics, which include a life ring, rescue tube, shepherd's crook, and life preserver. The equipment should be kept in good working condition and ready for use at all times. For convenience, it should always be stored in the same place so everyone knows where it is, and it should never be used for play.

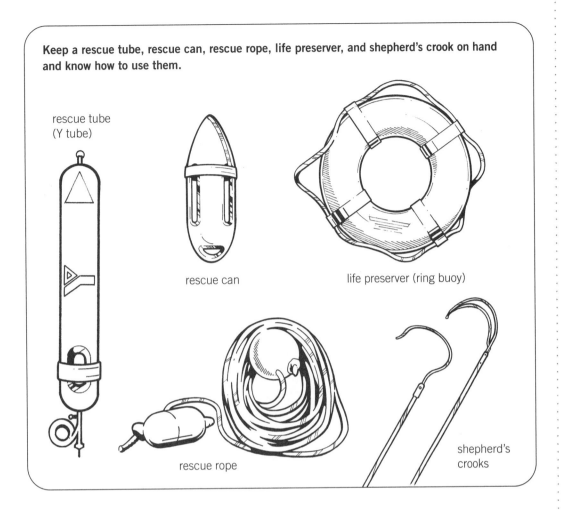

Keep a rescue tube, rescue can, rescue rope, life preserver, and shepherd's crook on hand and know how to use them.

rescue tube (Y tube)

rescue can

life preserver (ring buoy)

rescue rope

shepherd's crooks

Safety Accessories

It's always better to prevent an accident than to deal with one when it occurs. As you accessorize your pool and spa area, consider using some of these safety accessories:

~ Slip-resistant treads on ladders and steps
~ Clear signage that states the pool rules and advises against unsafe diving
~ Floating safety lines that mark the deep and shallow ends
~ Depth markers
~ An outdoor or cordless telephone, along with a list of emergency contacts and telephone numbers
~ For the adult supervisor, sunglasses to cut the glare off the water
~ Sunscreen to prevent sunburns
~ First-aid kit

POOL AND SPA DOS AND DON'TS

Pool and spa safety is serious business. But if everyone knows and obeys the rules, most accidents can be avoided. Though the list of safety rules could go on forever, here's a short list of dos and don'ts that everyone using your pool and spa, as well as those supervising the activities, should know about.

- ~ **DO** supervise children at all times.
- ~ **DO** make sure an adult is supervising the pool and spa area at all times. If he or she must leave the area for some reason, another supervisor should be appointed or all of the swimmers should exit the pool and spa until proper supervision can resume.
- ~ **DO** take children with you if you must leave the pool and spa area and no other adult is present to supervise, even if it's just for a few minutes.
- ~ **DON'T** allow anyone, regardless of age, to swim or bathe alone. Always use spotters or employ the buddy system.
- ~ **DO** teach children to swim, but don't assume that because they can swim they no longer require constant supervision. The best time to start swimming lessons is when your child is between 3 and 5 years old.
- ~ **DO** insist that poor swimmers stay in the shallow area. Mark the shallow area with a floating safety line across the pool.
- ~ **DON'T** leave floating toys in the pool or spa. They can attract young children, who may fall into the water trying to retrieve them.
- ~ **DON'T** allow children to play with tricycles and other wheeled toys near a pool or in-ground spa. A child could more easily fall into the water while playing with such toys.
- ~ **DON'T** allow swimmers to play between the pool wall and the ladder, where they may become trapped.
- ~ **DON'T** rely on inflatable toys or armbands to safeguard children. Always provide adult supervision even when using such items.
- ~ **DO** maintain a clean pool and spa at all times. Water that is cloudy or covered with leaves or algae can obstruct the view of swimmers.
- ~ **DO** use underwater lighting in the pool and spa at night so that the bottom is clearly visible.
- ~ **DO** make sure that all doors and gates leading to the pool and spa area have self-closing and self-latching devices that cannot be reached by small children. During periods when the pool or spa is unsupervised, make sure all doors and gates leading to the area are locked to prevent unauthorized entry.

- **DO** install around your pool or spa a fence, wall, or other barrier that's designed to discourage climbing and cannot be squeezed through by small children. Never leave objects (such as chairs or tables) near the barrier that children could use to help them climb into the pool and spa area.

- **DO** consider using an ASTM International (formerly known as the American Society for Testing and Materials) locking safety cover whenever the pool is not in use. Safety covers should be removed completely when the pool is being used so that swimmers don't become trapped under the cover. Use a tapered cover that allows rainwater to drain off the cover. Any standing water atop the cover should be removed to avoid the danger of pets or small children slipping on the cover and drowning in the collected water.

- **DON'T** dive into an aboveground pool.

- **DON'T** dive into a pool except from a diving board.

- If the pool has a diving board, **DON'T** dive deep and perpendicular to the water surface. Rather, dive shallow and direct your body upward as soon as you enter the water. Studies have shown that water alone does not slow down many divers enough for them to avoid hitting their heads on the pool bottom. What typically happens when your head hits a hard surface — even at slow speeds — is that your chin goes down to your chest. Though your head stops moving, the rest of your body doesn't, and the force can injure your neck, back, and/or spinal cord.

- **DON'T** run and dive, which can cause you to enter the water too fast and too far into the pool.

- **DON'T** attempt back dives in backyard pools, which aren't designed for this activity.

- **DON'T** go headfirst down a pool slide unless it's in deep water and you know how to steer up when you enter the water. This activity poses the same danger as diving.

- **DON'T** go down a slide backward.

- **DO** detach or secure your aboveground pool ladder when the pool is not in use to prevent unauthorized entry.

- **DO** inspect pool and spa ladders, handrails, and other fixtures periodically to make sure they are mounted securely.

- **DON'T** use a pool or spa that has a missing or broken grate over a drain. Swimmers' legs and arms can easily become entrapped in exposed drainpipes. Also, periodically inspect the inlet and outlet fittings, grates, skimmer, and main drain covers to make sure they're in good condition and can't be removed without tools. All swimmers, especially children, should be told not to play with these devices. People with long hair should not swim near outlets, where the suction can cause their hair to become tangled in the fitting, resulting in entrapment.

~ **DON'T** allow children to cry for help unless they truly need it.

~ **DO** keep lifesaving equipment near the pool where it's easily accessible.

~ **DO** install a phone or keep a cordless telephone near the pool or spa for use in an emergency. Along with the phone, have a list of emergency contact names and numbers. It's also a good idea to have your own address on the list in case a guest or someone unfamiliar with your address is making the call.

~ **DO** become trained in CPR (cardiopulmonary resuscitation).

~ **DON'T** use electrical devices (such as radios and CD players) where they could fall into the water. Whenever possible, use battery-operated appliances instead. Make sure all outside electrical outlets are equipped with a GFCI (ground fault circuit interrupter) to protect against electrical shock.

~ **DON'T** use glassware around pools and spas. Broken glass poses a serious danger to barefoot bathers and is nearly impossible to remove from the water. Instead, use plastic or paper cups and dishes.

~ **DO** instruct swimmers to shower before entering the pool or spa to remove dead skin, lotions, body oils, deodorants, and other contaminants that could quickly render your water sanitizer less effective.

~ **DON'T** allow people with infections or open wounds to use the pool or spa.

~ **DON'T** allow people — especially kids in diapers — to swim or bathe if they have diarrhea. Fecal matter can contaminate the water and infect others with any number of waterborne germs. Also, swimmers should wash their hands with soap and water after using the toilet or changing diapers so that germs don't make their way to the pool and spa.

~ **DON'T** mix alcohol or drug consumption with swimming or spa bathing. Alcohol and drugs can impair your judgment and lead you to engage in dangerous activities, such as diving into shallow water. In fact, studies show that alcohol is a factor in 50 to 80 percent of diving accidents. To avoid such risks, plan your pool or hot tub party so that the swimming comes before any drinking.

~ **DON'T** permit any horseplay that could lead to injury. Examples include throwing people into the pool and attempting to dive through inner tubes. No activity is 100 percent safe, but common sense will tell you which activities are less likely to result in injury.

- **DON'T** permit running around the pool deck, where slippery surfaces can cause people to fall.

- **DON'T** swim or soak during lightning or rainstorms because of the threat of electrocution if lighting were to strike the water.

- **DO** install a deck with a nonslip surface and keep the deck clear of debris at all times to help prevent slips and falls. Do check your deck periodically for cracks, chips, or other damage that may require fixing.

- **DO** post signs that outline the safety rules for your pool and spa. All aboveground pools and all shallow in-ground pools should have legible "No Diving" signs prominently displayed.

- **DON'T** allow spa water to exceed 104°F (40°C). In that temperature, limit use to just 15 minutes. Soaking too long may result in dizziness, lightheadedness, and fainting. Longer sessions can be spent in cooler water, or you may choose to exit the water and cool down before taking another soak. Use a reliable thermometer to monitor the water temperature at all times.

- **DO** consult a doctor before using a spa if you have a history of heart disease, diabetes, high or low blood pressure, or serious illness.

- **DON'T** use a hot tub if you are pregnant.

- **DON'T** use a hot tub if it is cloudy or has a strong chlorine smell. These conditions indicate that the water needs chemical treatment. Soaking in such water could result in a skin rash known as pseudomonas.

- **DO** exit a spa slowly, as the hot water may overly relax muscles and make you lightheaded.

THE DESIGNATED SUPERVISOR

Despite the wide range of safety products available, nothing can replace proper supervision of the pool or spa. This point has already been made, but it bears repeating. Sometimes, the more adults you have at a pool or spa event, the more lacking the supervision is. In fact, it's common for water-related accidents to occur even when several adults are present. That's because the adults assume that, with so many people around, someone else must be watching the children. The best way to avoid such tragedy is to appoint one individual whose sole responsibility is to supervise the pool activities. This person should be able to communicate the pool rules in a way that every swimmer understands, enforce them consistently, and know how to respond in an emergency situation. This person should not be asked to pour drinks for guests or flip burgers on the grill. If he or she must leave the pool area for some reason — even a short bathroom break — another supervisor should be named in the meantime.

FOR MORE INFORMATION

For more information on swimming pool and spa safety, contact the following organizations.

Centers for Disease Control (CDC)

The CDC offers health information on diseases and bacteria related to swimming pools and spas. www.healthyswimming.org

National Safety Council (NSC)

NSC is a national advocate for safety and health. The council offers fact sheets on water safety. www.nsc.org

National Spa & Pool Institute (NSPI)

An association for pool and spa professionals, NSPI develops safety standards and offers safety information for pool and spa owners. www.nspi.org

National Swimming Pool Foundation (NSPF)

NSPF is a nonprofit organization that promotes education and research to enhance safety in aquatic activities. www.nspf.com

U.S. Consumer Product Safety Commission (CPSC)

CPSC is a division of the U.S. government charged with protecting the public against unreasonable risks of injuries associated with consumer products. It offers recall information when necessary and provides safety information related to swimming pools and spas. www.cpsc.gov (search for key words *pools* and *spas*)

Repairs and Renovations

If you take good care of your pool and spa and keep the water balanced at all times, you can expect years of trouble-free enjoyment. But eventually there will come a time when you need to renovate — and that time may be sooner rather than later if you aren't diligent about water chemistry, if you accidentally damage the surface, or if natural disaster strikes and you have structural damage to the pool shell.

With the exception of repairing a small hole in a vinyl liner, repainting a pool, or fixing some loose tiles along the waterline, most repairs need to be undertaken by a trained professional — especially when the repair is really better described as a renovation.

There are a lot of reasons to renovate a pool. While some pool owners renovate out of necessity, others may simply want a new look in their backyard. People often renovate their kitchens and bathrooms because they want an updated design, and the same rationale often applies to pool owners who, for example, are looking to trade up their "plain-Jane," kidney-shaped pool with a concrete deck for a free-form lagoon-style pool with real boulders around the coping. Such a major overhaul of a pool requires the engineering and construction know-how of a skilled pool builder.

Whether you decide to call in the pros or wing it yourself, this chapter will give you a basic understanding of what's involved in some of the most common repairs and renovations. More detailed advice for your particular situation can be obtained from manufacturers or professional pool builders.

PLASTER SURFACES

If a plaster pool develops a stain, you might be able to remove it with one of the many stain-removal products available at pool and spa supply stores. But if the surface is heavily stained in many spots — whether from chemicals, minerals, or dirt — it may be time for a professional acid wash.

An acid wash strips away a tiny layer of plaster, exposing unblemished plaster beneath. Therefore, acid-wash only when it's really necessary. Otherwise you'll accelerate the need to replaster your pool and spa.

Acid is a highly toxic substance, and a complete acid wash of a pool should be undertaken by a professional technician, who will be trained in proper acid-washing techniques and the types of protective clothing and breathing apparatus needed, as well as the proper disposal guidelines for the used acid. You can expect to pay about $500 to acid-wash an average residential pool.

If you don't want to undertake an acid-wash, you might also consider fiberglassing or painting your plaster pool.

FIBERGLASS SURFACES

Fiberglass pool shells are a lot more durable today than they were years ago. Blistering and delaminating occur much less frequently, and fiberglass remains one of the easier surfaces to clean and maintain. Fiberglass shells have been known to crack, stain, and fade, however. Though minor chips, cracks, and blemishes can be repaired, you might need to re-fiberglass the entire shell if the situation is bad enough.

Fiberglass needs to be applied with precision and under the right environmental conditions in order to ensure a successful application. You should hire a trained professional to do this for you. If you can't find one in the Yellow Pages, your pool dealer should be able to refer you to one.

If your fiberglass pool is dingy but you don't want to re-fiberglass it, you could also consider painting it.

VINYL-LINED SURFACES

Small holes or tears in a vinyl liner can be repaired by anyone with handy tendencies, often without draining the water. Vinyl-repair kits are available from pool dealers. They include vinyl patches and underwater adhesive. To patch the liner, you simply cut a circular patch of vinyl that's large enough to overlap the hole by 1 inch (2.5 cm), apply adhesive, and then press the patch firmly over the hole.

If you hire a professional to do the job, he or she may use a heat gun to "weld" a vinyl patch in place. The heat-gun method should be used only by a trained professional because it's easy to melt the vinyl and cause more damage. The benefit of using a professional is that he or she may have access to vinyl swatches that closely match your original vinyl pattern. If not, he or she may still be able to mimic the pattern using special vinyl inks and some artistry.

The only way to fix major damage to a vinyl liner is to replace the entire liner. Under optimal conditions, a vinyl liner can be expected to last 5 to 10 years. But if the liner, especially the area above the waterline, is exposed to sun, it will fade and become brittle over time. The only solution in such a case is a new liner.

Installing a new liner is a task best left to a professional. Manufacturers can make custom liners to fit any pool size and shape, but the fit will be only as good as the measurements you provide the manufacturer. Expert help is invaluable in taking exact measurements of your pool. Also, professional installers can make sure that the new liner is set properly. They'll use vacuums to pull the liner snug against the floor and walls, increasing your chances for a wrinkle-free installation, and the proper tools to cut liners around skimmers, light niches, main drains, and other pool fittings.

EXTENDING THE LIFE OF A VINYL LINER

To help extend the life of your liner, follow these maintenance guidelines:

- Maintain the proper water balance. A low pH, especially below 7.0, may cause the liner to wrinkle.

- Maintain the proper sanitizer residual. If algae and bacteria are allowed to grow, they may cause stains on the liner. If the sanitizer level is too high, however, the liner may wrinkle.

- Do not use large, single doses of hydrochloric acid or muriatic acid to adjust pH or total alkalinity. If it's not blended carefully with the water, it might damage the liner's print pattern.

- Use a stain preventive to keep metals from staining the liner.

- To avoid possible bleaching of the liner caused by a reaction between different chemicals, allow one chemical to completely circulate throughout the pool before adding a second chemical.

- Clean the waterline regularly with a vinyl liner cleaner to keep dirt and grime from building up. Don't use household cleaners, which may damage the liner.

- Don't drain a vinyl-lined pool for any reason without consulting a pool professional first. The liner may shrink in an empty pool and not stretch back into shape without ripping or wrinkling.

POOL PAINT

Paints or coatings, as they're commonly referred to, are one of the cheapest options for restoring the look of a worn-out concrete, plaster, or fiberglass pool. In fact, painting can cost one third as much as replastering. Plus, with a wide-ranging palette of colors, paint allows you to nicely blend your old pool into a new landscape or create artistic designs on the walls and bottom. But don't fool yourself into thinking that painting a pool is as simple as painting the walls in your living room. There are many steps involved, and you need nearly perfect conditions to ensure professional results.

There are several types of pool paint, each with its unique advantages and disadvantages. The most common are epoxy, chlorinated rubber, and water-based acrylic.

Epoxy Coatings

Epoxy coatings are the most durable, lasting five to eight years. They provide a smooth, tile-like finish, and they resist chemicals, stains, abrasion, and algae. Epoxy coatings can be applied thickly, which is valuable if your plaster surface has been repeatedly acid-washed and is thinning out.

Epoxies come as two components, a base and a catalyst, which are mixed together prior to application. As soon as the two parts are mixed, the coating begins to cure. Thus, it has a "pot life" that is determined by the specific ingredients and the ambient temperature. You may have only a couple of hours to apply an epoxy, so never mix up more than you can apply in the given time frame.

Epoxy coatings are prone to chalking if they're not mixed or applied properly. Chalking can also occur as the coating ages. Though the chalking might cloud up the water when rubbed, it's not harmful to swimmers, according to manufacturers.

Epoxies are the best paints or coatings for fiberglass pools because they bond extremely well with fiberglass.

Chlorinated Rubber Coatings

Chlorinated rubber is the traditional coating for pools, and most painted pools use this type of coating. Chlorinated rubber is easy to apply and offers a durable, chemical-resistant coating with superior adhesion qualities. Though the paint can't be applied up as thickly as epoxy, it does chemically bond with previous paint coats, making it ideal for recoating surfaces previously painted with chlorinated rubber. Pools painted with chlorinated rubber coatings usually need to be repainted every three years or so.

Be advised that if chlorinated rubber is applied to a hot pool surface or in very hot weather, the paint dries too quickly and bubbles form in the surface. Once a second coat is applied, the solvents eat through the first coat as part of the bonding process, which causes the paint to pop off where the bubbles formed on the first coat.

Water-Based Acrylic Coatings

Water-based acrylic paint is the "new kid on the block" and not as popular as epoxy and chlorinated rubber coatings. The advantages of water-based acrylic paints are that they can be applied over damp surfaces and they clean up easily with soap and water. They are also colorfast, UV-resistant, and cheaper than other paints.

Choosing the Right Pool Paint

Before you prepare to paint your pool, make sure you have the right coating for the job. Not all paints can be applied over other types of paints. Use this chart to help you decide which paint is ideal for your particular pool and spa.

	EPOXY	CHLORINATED RUBBER	ACRYLIC
Previously Unpainted Pools			
Pool type:			
Concrete	***	***	***
Plaster	***	***	***
Fiberglass	***	NR	NR
Gunite	***	NR	NR
Previously Painted Pools			
Original paint:			
Epoxy	***	NR	*
Chlorinated rubber	NR	***	***
Acrylic	NR	NR	***
Physical Attributes			
Attribute:			
Ease of application	*	**	***
Chemical resistance	***	**	*
Stain resistance	***	***	*
Life expectancy	***	**	*

NR = not recommended; * = good; ** = better; *** = best.

On the negative side, because acrylic paints are often a flat finish, they stain more easily than other coatings. Also, water-based acrylics don't have the life span of the other coatings, so you can expect to paint every year if you use them.

Guidelines for Painting

After you've decided which paint is best for your particular situation, follow the manufacturer's instructions for preparing the surface and applying the paint. The following tips may help.

- Before painting, scrub the entire pool with trisodium phosphate. This removes dirt, oils, loose paint, and chalk. It will also help expose any surface problems that need to be addressed, such as cracks. If you do patch any holes or cracks, make sure the patch is cured before continuing with the next step.
- Before painting, mask off any areas you don't want painted; remove any drains, inlets, lights, and other fixtures; and protect the pool deck with drop cloths.
- Make sure you mix the paint thoroughly. If you're using several cans, mix them together to ensure you get the same shade and hue across the entire pool.
- Paint the walls first and the floor last. It may seem obvious, but be sure to paint the floor section near a ladder or steps last so that you can work your way out of the pool and not find yourself painted into a corner.
- Most manufacturers recommend a ⅜-inch roller for applying paint. Anything larger may leave behind hairs or allow air to become trapped beneath the paint as it's applied. For larger pools, you might want to use an airless spray gun.
- Etch the surface with a 15 to 20 percent solution of muriatic acid. This removes mineral deposits and stains. Some manufacturers recommend rewashing with trisodium phosphate after etching and thoroughly rinsing the surface with fresh water.

Acid-washing and acid etching produce dangerous fumes. When you acid-wash or acid-etch, make sure there is adequate ventilation in and around the pool. Wear a safety mask, safety goggles, rubber gloves, and a protective apron when working with these harsh chemicals. Also, when mixing acid, always add acid to water, and not vice versa. Pouring water into acid can cause an explosion.

- Apply paint when it's 50 to 90°F (10–32°C) outside, and work in the shade when possible, not in direct sunlight. Direct sunlight can start the paint drying from the outside, sealing in the solvent, which can then expand and cause the paint to blister. If necessary, rent a party tent that you can erect over the pool to create shade.

- If you're using epoxy or chlorinated rubber coatings, allow the final coat to dry fully. This could take several days with no rain. To determine if the surface is dry, tape a square of plastic wrap to each of the walls and leave it for a few hours. If you come back and see moisture condensing on the plastic wrap, the paint is not dry. Retest daily until no moisture is present on the plastic.

- With the exception of epoxy, apply paint in thin layers and allow it to dry to the touch before adding additional coats. With epoxy paints, however, additional coats need to be applied within 24 hours to ensure a proper chemical cure.

- If blistering occurs, scrape the area with a paint scraper or sand with #100-grit sandpaper. Then repaint.

- When painting steps, sprinkle a fine mist of sandbox sand over the first layer while it's still tacky. This creates a nonslip surface for swimmers entering or exiting the pool.

LEAKS AND CRACKS

Changes in temperature and settling earth can cause even a durable structure like a concrete pool to crack. If your concrete or gunite pool has a crack that's leaking water, you'll want to repair it immediately. Depending on the severity of the crack and your comfort level with this type of work, you might want to call in the professionals. Otherwise, feel free to attempt it yourself.

The Evaporation Test

Before you conclude you have a leak, make sure you're not just experiencing heavy evaporation caused by hot temperatures and high winds. Here's a simple test you can perform. Fill a 5-gallon bucket with water and place it next to your pool. Use a grease pencil or some other marking device that won't mar the pool to mark the level of the water in the pool and in the bucket. If the water level is decreasing due to evaporation alone, the water level the next day should have dropped the same amount in the pool and the bucket. If the water level in the pool has dropped more than it has in the bucket, you can assume you have a leak.

Finding the Leak

Of course, determining you have a leak is often easier than finding the leak. You may need to seek the help of trained professionals if your leak isn't obvious.

To save time and money, look at the most obvious places where a leak would occur. Around the equipment pad is a good place to start. Check for leaky valves and fittings and worn O-rings. Follow the plumbing lines to the pool while looking for wet spots on the ground.

If a leak is not noticeable upon visual inspection, you'll need to probe more deeply. A good test to home in on the leak is the pump on/pump off test. With the pump on, measure the amount of water lost during a 24-hour period, then do the same with the pump off. Compare the results. If the amount of water lost with the pump on is greater than the loss with the pump off, the leak is likely on the pressure side of the plumbing. If the loss with the pump on is less than the loss with the pump off, then the leak might be on the suction side. However, if there is no difference with the pump on or off, the leak may be in the pool shell.

In the pool shell, look for cracks or other damage along the tile line, around the skimmer, at light niches, and at all other openings. A common technique for finding leaks within the pool shell is a dye test, whereby colored dye is injected, usually with a syringe or dropper, around fixtures, cracks, or other areas suspected of leaking. If a leak is present, the dye will flow toward it.

Though you might be able to locate and fix a leak in the pool shell, an underground pipe leak is not so obvious or easy to repair. Some underground plumbing leaks are evident by soggy or settling ground around the pool area; others can only be detected by professionals using special listening devices, infrared thermography, fiberscopes, and other specialty equipment. Regardless, any leak that involves excavation to fix it is one for the professionals.

Repairing a Concrete Shell

You might be able to fix a leak in a concrete pool shell. You'll need safety goggles, a dust mask, a hammer, a chisel, a wire brush, hydraulic cement, a masonry pail, a wooden paddle and a trowel, gloves, a scraper, a hose, and masonry coating.

First, drain the pool. Don safety goggles and dust mask. Then use a hammer and chisel to enlarge the cracks or holes until they are at least ¾ inch deep and wide. Undercut — cutting more away from the bottom than from the top — as you work so the patching cement can be locked in. Remove all loose materials from the crack, then scrub and clean the area with a wire brush.

Mix the patching material according to package directions. Be sure to make only as much as you can use within the curing time. Put on your gloves and roll the patching material until it stiffens and becomes warm. Press the cement into the hole, beginning at the top, and keep pressure on the patch until the cement sets. Smooth the surface with a trowel and water. Some cements need to be kept moist for a specified period of time while they cure; see the manufacturer's instructions for details.

When you have patched all holes and cracks, waterproof the surface with masonry coating. Then prepare the surface for plastering or painting.

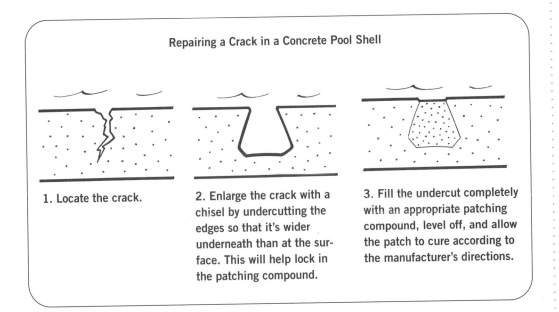

Repairing a Crack in a Concrete Pool Shell

1. Locate the crack.

2. Enlarge the crack with a chisel by undercutting the edges so that it's wider underneath than at the surface. This will help lock in the patching compound.

3. Fill the undercut completely with an appropriate patching compound, level off, and allow the patch to cure according to the manufacturer's directions.

Appendixes

A. POOL MAINTENANCE SCHEDULE

Diligent, consistent care of your pool is the best way to ensure a safe and healthy swimming environment. Though every pool is different because of location, design, and bather load, some general maintenance guidelines will apply. For a maintenance schedule customized for your particular pool, contact your pool builder or service technician. In the meantime, follow these steps.

Daily

~ Check the water level and fill to recommended level.
~ Test pH and sanitizer levels and make needed adjustments.
~ Empty skimmer basket and pump strainer basket.
~ Skim leaves and other debris from pool surface.
~ Circulate the water until it turns over at least once — about eight hours.

Weekly

~ Brush all pool walls and floor to prevent algae buildup.
~ Clean waterline tile or vinyl.
~ Vacuum the pool bottom.
~ Shock the water in the evening. (Additional shocking may be needed after a rainstorm, heavy bather load, or exceptionally hot weather.)
~ Add an algaecide the day after you shock the water.

Monthly

~ Clean or backwash the filter. More frequent filter cleaning may be necessary depending on how much debris is introduced into the pool.
~ Test water for total alkalinity, calcium hardness, and stabilizer levels.

Mid-Season

~ Clean cartridge filters to remove any oils and dirt that have accumulated.

If you're having difficulty balancing the water, bring a sample to your pool supply dealer for professional testing and analysis. A proper water sample should include at least 8 ounces retrieved from at least 18 inches below the surface, preferably from the deep end. Store the sample in a clean plastic container and take it immediately to your dealer for testing.

B. HOW TO INSTALL AN ABOVEGROUND POOL

A professional pool installer could charge $500 to $1,000 to install your aboveground pool, depending on the size and style of the pool and how much site preparation needs to be done. If you feel up to the task, you might be able to install the pool yourself over a weekend with the help of a few other willing souls. The following guidelines should help. (Note that some of the procedures may differ depending on the type of pool you buy.)

1. Read the Instructions

Read the manufacturer's installation instructions before you begin work. If you have any questions, contact the manufacturer or the dealer from whom you purchased the pool. Your careful attention to the instructions will not only ensure a proper installation but also prevent you from mishandling the equipment in a way that voids the manufacturer's warranty.

2. Locate Buried Utility Lines

Many communities offer free "dig-safe" hotlines you can call to schedule an appointment for someone to visit your home and mark where utility lines are buried. If you don't call and you happen to hit a utility line during excavation, you most likely will be liable for the cost of repairs to the line.

3. Obtain Necessary Permits

Obtain any building permits you might need. Also check out any zoning laws that may apply to the type of pool you're going to install.

4. Select a Site

The ideal installation site provides drainage away from the pool and is not near any overhead electrical wires. If possible, keep the pool away from trees, which will dump leaves and debris into the pool water. Make sure the site provides easy access to an electrical supply so that you can power the pool equipment. If you have a septic system, don't place the pool over it.

Once you've chosen a site, mark it out with stakes and then use string and spray paint to denote the perimeter of the pool. To find the perimeter of a round pool, place a stake in the center of the site and rotate a radius-length string around it.

5. Excavate

Excavate a level base. The rule of thumb is to dig from high ground to low ground so that you don't have to fill in any areas later. Some manufacturers recommend leveling an area that extends 3 feet past the perimeter of the pool on all sides. Make sure all protruding rocks, roots, and debris are removed from the leveled area.

To save time, you might want to rent a sod cutter, which will remove the sod in nice rows that can be transplanted elsewhere. If you're attempting to level a sloping lawn, you also may want to rent a front-end loader or Bobcat, which will help you accomplish in minutes what it would take hours to complete with hand shovels.

Though being ½ inch out of level most likely won't have a negative effect, you should strive for perfect level. The best tool for leveling the ground is a surveyor's transit. Without one, you could use a *straight* 2x4 board with a level set on top of it.

6. Assemble the Bottom Rim and Wall Supports

Assemble the pool walls, following the manufacturer's instructions. You'll begin by laying out the bottom rim. Drive stakes every few feet around the outside of the rim to keep it from shifting as you begin to put up the walls.

After the rim is set, create a stable foundation for the upright supports by burying a 16-by-16-inch patio block so that it is flush with the ground at each spot where an upright support will be located. Make sure that all of the supports are level with each other. This is also a good time to take some measurements to make sure the pool frame is square.

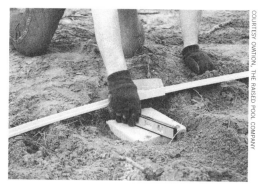

Cover the leveled area with non-translucent black polyethylene to keep roots from growing up through the vinyl liner.

Patio blocks are placed level in the ground where the upright supports will go.

7. Assemble the Walls

Note where you plan to install the equipment, and start the pool wall in the center of the base plate to the left of the future equipment pad. The pool wall should be rolled up and standing upright as you begin inserting it into the track. It will take several people to support the heavy pool wall and help guide it into the track. To keep the wall from falling over, you may want to stabilize it with S-hooks hung over the top of the wall and tied to stakes around the pool's exterior, like a tent. If you tape the ends of the S-hooks, they shouldn't scratch the pool wall.

After the wall has been completely unrolled and installed in the track, the bolt holes along the two ends should align. If they don't, you'll need to slightly adjust the rim frame until they do. Install and tighten the bolts, then file down any burrs on the bolt heads and cover the seam with several layers of duct tape to prevent possible damage to the liner.

At this point, check to make sure the pool is level at several points. If it's out of level more than 1 inch, you'll need to dismantle the pool and re-level the bottom.

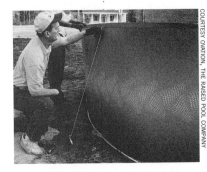

The wall is stabilized with S-hooks and stakes to keep it from falling in.

The Wind Factor

You'll have a hard time erecting the pool walls if the wind is any stronger than a very mild breeze. The big wall pieces catch the wind much like sails, dragging their "boat" — you and whoever else is holding on to them — with them. So wait for a calm day before trying to install the pool walls.

---

8. Prepare the Floor

Rake the sand floor to a depth of 2 inches and form the wall cove — the transitional curve from the floor to the wall — according to the installation manual. The cove ensures that the pool doesn't contain any sharp corners, which are difficult to clean and could stress the liner.

Dampen the sand floor and compact it with a drum roller. Brush out any lines and footprints with a medium-bristle push broom. For an ultra-smooth floor finish, the dampened sand can be hand-troweled.

9. Hang the Liner

If possible, install the liner when the temperature is above 70°F (21°C). The warm weather will make the liner more flexible and less likely to wrinkle. Carefully unfold the liner and lift it over the wall and into the pool. Make sure the print side is up and the shiny side is down. Avoid dragging the liner across the sand bottom, which will destroy the careful leveling work you did in the previous step. Instead, gently pull it into place. Make sure the seams are straight. If you have an oval or circular pool, make sure the bottom seam matches the circumference of the pool. Smooth out the liner, working any extra material toward the wall edge.

Some liners hang over the walls, while others have a beaded edge that fits into a track on the walls. Follow the manufacturer's instructions for the type of liner you have. Some installers suggest using a shop vacuum to suck the air out from between the pool shell and liner, helping remove wrinkles and set the liner. The vacuum hose can be fed through the skimmer opening.

10. Install the Uprights and Top Rail

Depending on the type of pool you have, the uprights should be installed either before or while the pool is filled with water. Consult your owner's manual for the proper installation sequence for your pool.

Connect the uprights to the base plate at the bottom and at the top with the top rail. Use a carpenter's level to ensure the uprights are plumb. Loosely fasten the top rail as you work your way around the pool, then go back and tighten all of the screws once everything is in place. Some pools have parts that snap together, greatly reducing the amount of hardware needed to secure the pool.

11. Fill the Pool

Tape a soft cloth to the end of the hose you'll be using to fill the pool so the metal doesn't damage the liner. Start filling the pool slowly; increase the water flow as the liner stretches and the wrinkles come out. To speed up the process, especially if your water pressure is low, you might want to hire a water truck to deliver water to the site.

When the pool water is about 16 inches deep, measure the distance from the top of the water to the top of the pool at various points around the pool. If the distances among the points vary more than 1 inch, the pool should be drained and the structure re-leveled. Turn off the water when the water level is just below the skimmer opening.

12. Install Pool Equipment

Install the equipment according to the manufacturer's instructions. You'll need to cut holes in the liner where the skimmer and inlet fittings go. Make sure the equipment is placed on level, dry ground — preferably on a concrete pad or a bed of patio blocks.

Install all safety decals and signs that came with your pool, indicating "no diving" and other safety measures.

Install the pool ladder according to the assembly instructions. If the ladder is an A-frame design, you may want to install it early and use it to enter and exit the pool shell while you're setting up the walls and forming the sand floor.

13. Balance the Water

Balance and sanitize the water. See chapter 4 for more information.

C. RESOURCES

Whether you're looking for help constructing a pool, tips for improving your aquatic workout, a professional dealer in your area, or ways to make your pool and spa safer, these resources can help.

Aquatic Exercise

Aquatic Exercise Association (AEA)
P.O. Box 1609, Nokomis, FL 34274-1609; phone: 888-AEA-WAVE
Web: www.aeawave.com

Aquatic Therapy & Rehab Institute, Inc.
3650-A Centre Circle, Fort Mill, SC 29715; phone: 803-802-5400
Web: www.atri.org

Arthritis Foundation
P.O. Box 7669, Atlanta, GA 30357-0669; phone: 800-283-7800
Web: www.arthritis.org

Human Kinetics
P.O. Box 5076, Champaign, IL 61825-5076; phone: 800-747-4457
Web: www.humankinetics.com
A publisher of fitness books, including such titles as Aquatic Exercise Toolbox, Fitness Aquatics, Water Exercise, Water Fitness After 40, Water Fun and Fitness, *and* Fantastic Water Workouts.

United States Water Fitness Association (USWFA)
P.O. Box 3279, Boynton Beach, FL 33424; phone: 561-732-9908
Web: www.uswfa.com

International Swimming Hall of Fame (ISHOF)
One Hall of Fame Drive, Fort Lauderdale, FL 33316; phone: 954-462-6536
Web site: www.ishof.org
Honoring those who have distinguished themselves in swimming, diving, water polo, and synchronized swimming. ISHOF is a nonprofit educational organization that maintains efforts for safety among numerous water sources — from pools and spas to oceans and streams.

Construction and Safety

American National Standards Institute (ANSI)
25 West 43rd Street, New York, NY 10036; phone: 212-642-4900
Web site: www.ansi.org
A private, nonprofit organization that coordinates the development of private-sector voluntary standards. Among the ANSI standards concerning the spa and pool industry are six sets of guidelines developed by the National Spa and Pool Institute for the design, equipment, installation, and use of spas and pools.

American Society for Testing & Materials (ASTM)

100 Barr Harbor Drive, West Conshohocken, PA 19428; phone: 610-832-9585
Fax: 610-832-9555
Web site: www.astm.org
ASTM is primarily a standards-development agency that establishes testing methods. Among its standards is F-1346 for pool and spa safety covers.

American Society of Mechanical Engineers (ASME)

22 Law Drive, Fairfield, NJ 07007; phone: 800-843-2763, 973-882-1167
Web site: www.asme.org
ASME develops standards for such products as plumbing fixtures, general-purpose pipe threads, and suction fittings for use in pools and spas. The voluntary standards are often referenced in other standards and adopted in part or whole by code-writing groups, state building departments, and other jurisdictions. Though the society does not directly certify or endorse products, manufacturers can certify that they've met ASME design standards as a means to enhance the value of and confidence in their products.

California Redwood Association

405 Enfrente Drive, Suite 200, Novato, CA 94949; phone: 415-382-0662,
888-225-7339
Web site: www.calredwood.org
One of the oldest trade associations in the forest products industry. It promotes the use of redwood; provides technical services to manufacturers, specifiers, and builders; and maintains high product quality through its Redwood Inspection Service division.

California Spa & Pool Industry Education Council (SPEC)

980 Ninth Street, Suite 430, Sacramento, CA 95814; phone: 916-447-4113
Web site: www.calspec.org
A private, nonprofit organization, SPEC represents all segments of the swimming pool and spa industry in legislative and regulatory matters at the local, state, regional, and special district levels. The group has tackled such industry issues as mandatory water rationing for pools and spas, fencing regulations, construction bans and guidelines, contractor regulations, pool chemical use, and mandatory solar heating for pool and spa water with natural gas heater bans.

International Association of Plumbing & Mechanical Officials (IAPMO)

5001 E. Philadelphia Street, Ontario, CA 91761; phone: 909-472-4100
Web site: www.iapmo.org
Municipalities across the United States adopt IAPMO codes. Manufacturers' products are required to meet the codes in jurisdictions that choose to adopt the codes. Installers must follow all IAPMO guidelines.

International Conference of Building Officials Evaluation Service (ICBO ES)
5360 Workman Mill Road, Whittier, CA 90601-2299; phone: 888-699-0541
Web site: www.icboes.org
A nonprofit organization that promotes public safety by evaluating current and innovative construction technology for compliance with codes, standards, and acceptance criteria. Engineers, architects, manufacturers, designers, ICBO members, and the construction industry look to ICBO ES to provide verification that certain materials, systems, and equipment are acceptable alternatives or conform to standards specified in the codes.

United States Consumer Product Safety Commission (CPSC)
4330 East-West Highway, Bethesda, MD 20814; phone: 800-638-2772
Web site: www.cpsc.gov
With its power to recall products and set standards, this government agency serves consumers by investigating claims of unsafe products. In its role as product-safety watchdog, the group responds to consumer complaints and evaluates voluntary standards to determine if they provide sufficient levels of safety or if they should be replaced by mandatory standards.

Western Red Cedar Lumber Association (WRCLA)
1200-555 Burrard Street, Vancouver, BC V7X 1S7, Canada; phone: 604-684-0266
Web site: www.wrcla.org
A nonprofit trade association representing quality producers of western red cedar lumber products in British Columbia, Canada, and the U.S. Pacific Northwest states. Association members are dedicated to producing quality siding, decking, paneling, and other specialty cedar products in a wide range of sizes and grades. Collectively, these manufacturers annually produce 950 million board feet of cedar products. The WRCLA is dedicated to providing the construction industry with information about WRCLA member products, their specifications, and proper use.

Professional Groups and Associations

Associated Swimming Pool Industries of Florida (ASPI)
3701 N. Country Club Drive, Suite 2107, Aventura, FL 33180-1721;
phone: 305-937-0960
More than 30 years old, ASPI is a nonprofit organization of pool and spa professionals and allied businesses. The group uses its dues for ongoing reports on products, legislation, and regulatory rulings.

Independent Pool & Spa Service Association Inc. (IPSSA)
P.O. Box 15828, Long Beach, CA 90815; phone: 888-360-9505
Web site: www.ipssa.com
An organization serving pool and spa service technicians in Arizona, California, Nevada, and Texas. The group sponsors technical and business seminars, a monthly newsletter, and other services.

Master Pools Guild

9601 Gayton Road, Suite 207, Richmond, VA 23233-4963; phone: 800-392-3044
Web site: www.masterpoolsguild.com
An exclusive group of independent pool builders who build permanent pools and spas that incorporate the latest design techniques.

National Association of Professional Safety Cover Installers (NAPSCI)

1105 California N.E., Albuquerque, NM 87110; phone: 505-266-4662
NAPSCI promotes safety and professionalism in the pool cover industry. The organization verifies that its members are factory-trained service technicians and installers of safety covers for independently listed automatic and manual safety cover manufacturers. Each member must use covers that meet or exceed ASTM standards.

National Plasterers Council

21939 Camille Drive, Nuevo, CA 92567; phone: 909-928-1112
Web site: www.plasterscouncil.org
The National Plasterers Council is a group of pool plasterers who benefit from the organization's research and expertise. The council publishes a technical manual, hosts an annual conference, and publishes materials for consumers promoting the benefits of swimming pool plaster and information necessary to help them make educated decisions about work to be done on their swimming pools.

National Spa & Pool Institute (NSPI)

2111 Eisenhower Avenue, Alexandria, VA 22314; phone: 703-838-0083
Web site: www.nspi.org
NSPI is an umbrella organization for the spa and pool industry, representing the interests of manufacturers, manufacturers' representatives, distributors, builders, installers, basic materials suppliers, retailers, service companies, subcontractors, professional pool managers, independent pool service technicians, and other associated members or firms. The group also publishes pool and spa purchasing and safety information for consumers.

National Swimming Pool Foundation (NSPF)

P.O. Box 60701, Colorado Springs, CO 80961
Web site: www.nspf.com
A nonprofit organization dedicated to research and education in aquatic safety. The 33-year-old group serves swimming pool professionals and consumers worldwide. Its CPO course is a training program for the National Registration of Certified Pool-Spa Operators. CPOs are trained in the most advanced techniques in safety, water chemistry, maintenance, and management.

Professional Pool Operators of America (PPOA)

P.O. Box 164, Newcastle, CA 95658; phone: 916-663-1265
Web site: www.ppoa.org
PPOA serves operators of large swimming pools and waterparks. Its goal is the recognition, training, and refinement of the operators of institutional and public aquatic facilities throughout the Americas and the developed world.

United Pool & Spa Association (UPSA)
P.O. Box 13223, Jacksonville, FL 32206; phone: 904-353-4403
UPSA is a group for pool contractors, service companies, and pool supply stores in Florida. Members agree to the association's policy of fair and honest customer service, and all member pool builders must meet or exceed Florida's building codes.

Energy Resources

Department of Energy (DOE)
Forrestal Building, 1000 Independence Avenue S.W., Washington, DC 20585;
phone: 202-586-5575
Web site: www.energy.gov
The DOE sets minimum energy-efficiency standards for fuel-fired pool heaters. The current energy-efficient requirement for gas-fired pool heaters is 78 percent, which means heaters must be at least 78 percent efficient to be sold legally in the United States. The DOE also encourages the use of pool covers and solar or high-efficiency heating systems through its Reducing Swimming Pool Energy Costs Program.

Federal Trade Commission (FTC)
600 Pennsylvania Avenue N.W., Suite 421, Washington, DC 20580;
phone: 202-326-2180
Web site: www.ftc.gov
The FTC has placed pool heaters on its list of appliances that must have yellow Energy Guide labels. The Energy Guide labeling system is related to the DOE's minimum energy-efficiency standards, but the two are separate. The DOE establishes the minimum and dictates how tests should be conducted; the FTC is concerned with whether products are labeled accurately.

GLOSSARY

Acid. A liquid or dry chemical used to lower the pH of pool and spa water.

Acid demand. The amount of acid required to lower an alkaline body of water's pH to neutral.

Acidic. Having a pH below neutral.

Acid-wash. To clean plaster with a solution of muriatic acid and water. Acid washing should be undertaken only by a trained pool and spa professional.

Aerator. A pipe vented to the atmosphere that allows air to be mixed with water. It is most commonly used in spas.

Air-relief valve. A valve on pool filters that allows trapped air to be discharged safely.

Air switch. A control device used to operate spa equipment safely. An air switch button, when pressed, sends air pressure along a plastic hose to an on/off switch, thereby keeping wet bathers safely away from electrical devices.

Algae. Microscopic plant life that grows in water and on underwater surfaces.
  Black alga. A type of alga that forms tough, dark-colored spots on pool surfaces; it is particularly visible in plaster pools.
  Green alga. A type of alga that grows in free-floating forms in the water and on pool walls; it is bright green.
  Mustard alga. A type of alga that grows on pool walls and is yellow, orange, or yellow-brown.

Algaecide. A chemical agent used to kill and prevent future growth of algae.

Algistat. A chemical that inhibits the growth of algae.

Alkaline. Having a pH above neutral; also, a chemical used to raise the pH of pool and spa water.

Alkalinity. The degree to which a substance is alkaline.

Alum. A flocculating agent that causes dirt and other suspended particles in water to group together so they can more easily be removed by the pool or spa's filter. Potassium alum and ammonium alum are the most common types.

Antivortex. The characteristic of a plumbing fixture that prevents a whirlpool effect, thereby eliminating the risk of entrapment. Main drain covers often have antivortex covers to prevent suction that could trap swimmers (or, particularly, their hair, if it's long).

Backwash. To reverse the flow direction of water in a filter to clean the filter of accumulated debris.

Bacteria. Single-celled, often parasitic microorganisms without distinct nuclei or organized cell structures. Various species are responsible for decay, fermentation, nitrogen fixation, and many plant and animal diseases.

Baking soda. *See* Sodium bicarbonate.

Balanced water. Water that is neither corrosive nor scaling, falling in the pH range of 7.2 to 7.8. Balanced water is achieved by proper adjustment of five factors: pH level, total alkalinity, calcium hardness, total dissolved solids, and temperature. These factors make available the mineral constituents that water requires as its "food." If the water has less than the required minerals, the water is "hungry" or corrosive (acidic), obtaining minerals from metals in pool equipment and from plaster or concrete. When water has more minerals than it requires (alkaline), the excess minerals are deposited onto pool surfaces and the interior of pipes and equipment as scale.

Base. An alkaline substance.

Basic. Another term for *alkaline*.

Bather load. The number of bathers or swimmers who use a spa or pool in a 24-hour period.

Bather occupancy. The number of bathers or swimmers in a spa or pool at a given time.

Bicarbonate of soda. *See* Sodium bicarbonate.

Bleed. To remove air from a pipe or piece of equipment, such as a filter, so water can fill the space.

Blower. An electromechanical device that generates air pressure and supplies air to spa jets and rings.

Bond beam. The top of a pool or spa wall, which is designed to be stronger than the rest of the wall because it must support coping and decking.

Bonding system. The wiring between electrical equipment and the ground to prevent electric shock in case of a faulty circuit.

Booster pump. A pump added to a pool or spa circulation system to create additional pressure for jets, water features, automatic pool cleaners, and other equipment.

British thermal unit (Btu). The amount of heat required to raise 1 pound of water 1 degree Fahrenheit.

Bromine. A chemical element used for water sanitization, particularly in hot tubs and spas. It's a member of the halogen family of compounds.

Btu. *See* British thermal unit.

Buffer. A substance that helps water resist changes in pH.

Burner tray. The component in the bottom of a gas heater that controls the burning of gas.

Calcium carbonate. A mineral that can precipitate out of water and form deposits on pool and spa surfaces. It's the major component of scale.

Calcium hardness. The mineral content of water. Water obtains minerals, primarily calcium and magnesium, from rocks and other solids over which it moves. The average hardness of surface waters in the United States varies from less than 60 ppm (parts per million) in the Northwest, Southeast, and Northeast to more than 240 ppm in some central states. Hardness is a disadvantage for household applications, but in pool water hardness helps protect pool surfaces from the corrosive effects of water.

Calcium hypochlorite. A granular form of chlorine generally produced in a compound of 70 percent chlorine and 30 percent inert materials.

Cartridge filter. A water filter that uses pleated polyester fabric as the filter medium. Cartridge filters can screen out particles larger than 10 to 20 microns.

Cavitation. Failure of a pump to move water because a vacuum, caused by the discharge capacity of the pump exceeding its suction ability, has been created.

Channeling. The formation of channels in sand of a sand filter, which allows water to pass through unfiltered.

Chelating agent. Chemical compound that prevents minerals in solution in a body of water from precipitating out of solution and depositing on the surfaces of a pool or spa.

Chemical feeder. A device used to feed (and sometimes meter) chemicals into a pool. Types include injection feeders, proportioning pumps, pot feeders, and dry feeders.

Chloramines. Chemical compounds formed when chlorine comes in contact with ammonia (from garden fertilizers, urine, or body sweat and oils). Chloramines are not effective as sanitizers; contact with them can result in burning eyes and skin irritation. They usually produce a strong chlorine odor. (Contrary to popular belief, eye irritation and a strong chlorine smell do not indicate that pool water has too much chlorine but, rather, that it has too many chloramines; in other words, it needs *more* chlorine.)

Chlorinator. A device that dispenses, regulates, and meters the amount of chlorine introduced into water on a semiautomatic or fully automatic basis.

Chlorine. An oxidizing chemical sanitizer widely used in pool and spa water purification. A member of the halogen family, chlorine kills algae and bacteria and oxidizes (burns up) suspended dirt particles in water. For use by pool owners, chlorine comes in several forms: liquid, granular, tablet, and stick.

Chlorine demand. The quantity of chlorine required to destroy pollutants in the pool (bacteria, algae, chloramines). Once this "demand" is satisfied, a small residual amount of free chlorine becomes available in the water to keep it in a sanitary condition.

Chlorine residual. The amount of active chlorine (also known as free chlorine or free available chlorine) available for sanitizing after the initial chlorine demand of the water has been met. Inactive chlorine forms chloramines.

Colorimetric. A type of chemical test in which reagents added to water change in color to reflect the presence of certain substances. The color is compared to a color chart (provided by the manufacturer of the test) to gauge the concentration of those substances.

Coping. The cap on the edge of a pool or spa.

Corona discharge. A type of ozone generator that produces ozone by passing electricity through oxygen and water. Ozone is used as a sanitizer.

Cyanuric acid. A mild acid of low toxicity with little effect on pH. It can be added to pool water to retard the loss of chlorine due to sunlight. Chlorinated isocyanurics are chlorine mixtures that contain cyanuric acid; they're called *stabilized chlorine*.

Diatomaceous earth (DE). A fine, powderlike substance consisting of the compressed, powdered skeletons of tiny prehistoric diatoms. DE is used as a filter medium (septum) for swimming pools. DE filters can screen out particles larger than 2 to 5 microns.

Dichlor. The full chemical name is sodium *dichlor*isocyanurate dihydrate. Dichlor is a stabilized chlorine donor usually sold in the form of granules of 55 to 60 percent available chlorine. When dissolved in water, it dissociates (splits up) into hypochlorous acid (free chlorine) and cyanuric acid.

Diethyl phenylene diamene (DPD). A chemical reagent used to detect the presence of free available chlorine in a body of water.

Diffuser. A housing inside a pump that covers the impeller, reducing the speed of the water while increasing pressure in the system to help eliminate airlock.

Distributor. The device used in a pool filter to divert incoming water and prevent erosion of the filter medium (for example, the sand in a sand filter).

DPD. *See* Diethyl phenylene diamene.

Dry acid. *See* Sodium bisulfate.

EDTA. *See* Ethylenediamine tetra-acetic acid.

Effluent. The water discharging from a pipe or equipment.

Electrolysis. An electron flow (migration of ions) between two dissimilar metals submerged in water, which causes corrosion.

Etching. Corrosion of a surface by water that is acidic or low in total alkalinity and/or calcium hardness.

Ethylenediamine tetra-acetic acid (EDTA). A reagent used for testing calcium hardness. The tester adds drops of EDTA, one at a time, into a solution until it turns blue. The number of drops required to turn the solution blue is compared to a chart to evaluate the hardness of the sample.

Expansion joint. The gap between the coping and the deck that permits expansion and contraction of the materials without damage.

Fiber-optic lighting. Underwater and landscape lighting that illuminates by sending light along a plastic fiber-optic cable from a remote illuminator.

Free chlorine. *See* Chlorine residual.

Filter. A device that strains impurities, dirt, and debris from spa and pool water. The filter is built into a pool or spa's circulation system.

Filter cycle. The length of time the filter operates before it needs to be backwashed or cleaned.

Flocculant. A compound, such as alum, that causes small particles of suspended dirt or other materials to clump together into larger masses.

Flow rate. Volume of flow per unit of time, usually expressed in gallons per minute (gpm).

Freeboard. The vacant vertical area between the top of the filter medium and the underside of the top of the filter.

Free available chlorine. *See* Chlorine residual.

Gasket. A material inserted between two connected objects to prevent leaks.

Gelcoat. A thin finishing coat of resin applied over fiberglass.

Ground fault circuit interrupter (GFCI). A built-in circuit breaker that protects against shock by shutting down a circuit or receptacle when it detects a problem.

Gunite. A dry mixture of cement and sand that is mixed with water and sprayed onto surfaces lined with steel reinforcing rods, thereby creating the shell of a pool or spa. The technical term for gunite is *pneumatically applied concrete.*

Halogens. A family of oxidizing agents that includes chlorine and bromine.

Hard water. Water is considered hard if its calcium hardness is more than 250 ppm (parts per million) and its alkalinity is more than 150 ppm. The pH of hard water tends to be relatively stable, but it may be best to use a mildly acidic type of chlorine, such as trichlor, to achieve a pH balance in the water.

Hardness. The amount of dissolved minerals (mostly calcium and magnesium) in water. High levels of these minerals in unbalanced water can cause scale and cloudy water. Low levels cause water to "attack" or corrode pool surfaces and equipment. High levels of calcium and magnesium in balanced water contribute to the protection of plaster and metals.

Head. The measurement of pressure (expressed in feet) in a water circulation system created by friction, resistance, distance, and lift.

Head-loss value. The amount of pressure, expressed in feet, that a component imposes on the water circulation system.

Heater. A device that raises the temperature of water using natural gas, electricity, propane, or solar or mechanical energy.

Heat exchanger. The copper tubing in a heater through which water flows, absorbing the rising heat from the burner below.

Heat pump. A type of pool and spa heater that extracts heat from ambient air and transfers it to the water.

High-rate sand filter. A filter that uses sand for the filtering medium. It's designed for flow rates greater than 5 gpm but less than 15 to 20 gpm per square foot. Sand filters can screen out particles larger than 20 to 40 microns.

Hopper. The deep, bowl-shaped portion of the pool near the main drain.

Horsepower (hp). A unit of measurement that refers to the strength of a mechanical device. One horsepower equals 746 watts (or the amount of power needed to move 550 pounds one foot in one second).

Hot tub. Another name for a spa. Generally, it refers to a spa set above the ground.

Hydrochloric acid (HCL). *See* Muriatic acid.

Hydrostatic pressure. The force created by underground water. If strong enough, it can force pools to pop out of the ground. Sometimes a hydrostatic check valve is placed in the pool's main drain to allow excessive groundwater into the pool.

Hypochlorite. Any salt form of hypochlorous acid (chlorine). For comparison's sake, household bleach has about 5 percent chlorine.
  Calcium hypochlorite. A powder or tablet form of chlorine that contains about 70 percent pure chlorine.
  Lithium hypochlorite. An organic, granular, highly soluble form of chlorine containing about 35 percent available chlorine.
  Sodium hypochlorite. The most common liquid form of chlorine for pool sanitizing. It contains about 16 percent chlorine. It disperses quickly in water and does not add to water hardness, but it does raise pH and alkalinity.

Hypochlorous acid (HOCL). A form of free chlorine formed when active chlorine is added to water.

Impeller. The rotating part of a pump that creates centrifugal force, or suction power.

Influent. Water entering the pool through a filter or other device.

Inlet. A fitting or port through which water passes into the pool.

Jet. An inlet fitting through which water returns to the spa or pool at a high velocity.

Kilowatt. A unit equal to 1,000 watts of electrical power. Electricity is sold by the kilowatt-hour, meaning a certain fee is charged for every 1,000 watts used.

Laterals. The horizontal filter grids at the bottom of a sand filter.

Leaf rake. An open net secured to a frame that attaches to a telepole; it's used to skim leaves and debris from the surface of water.

Main drain. The outlet or drain in the bottom of the deepest part of the pool, through which water is drawn to the circulating pump and filter.

Mottling. Shading, streaking, blotchiness, or other forms of uneven coloring on a surface, particularly plaster.

Multiport valve. A valve having three or more control positions for various filter operations.

Muriatic acid. A commercial form of hydrochloric acid. It's used to lower the pH of pool water and for etching and acid-washing pool surfaces.

Neutral. Describes a pH reading that is neither acidic nor alkaline. Neutral pH is 7 on a scale of 1 to 14.

O ring. A thin rubber gasket used to create a waterproof seal in certain plumbing joints or between two parts of a device, such as between the lid and the strainer pot on a pump.

Orothotolidine (OTO). A reagent used in a water test kit to measure the amount of residual or free chlorine present.

Outlet line. A pipe from the main drain and/or skimmers used to direct water from the pool to the pump and filter.

Overflow gutter. A gutter around the top of a pool that carries waste away from the surface water to the filter and catches water displaced by swimmers. Not all pools have an overflow gutter.

Oxidize. To burn up. In pool water, hypochlorous acid (chlorine) oxidizes algae, bacteria, and suspended dirt particles.

Ozone (O_3). An unstable sanitizer produced by an ozonator. Because it does not leave a residual, it cannot be used alone; it must be used in conjunction with a chemical sanitizer.

pH. The abbreviation for potential hydrogen. The pH scale ranges from 1 to 14 and indicates the acidity or alkalinity of pool water. A neutral solution has a measure of 7. Readings below 7 indicate an acidic condition; readings above 7 indicate an alkaline condition.

Phenol red (phenolsulfonephthalein). A chemical reagent used to measure the pH of water.

Pilot. The small gas flame that ignites the burner tray of a heater.

Plaster. A mixture of white or colored cement, aggregates, and additives that is applied to the shell of a gunite pool or spa to waterproof the shell and create an attractive surface.

Potassium monopersulfate. An oxidizing chemical used to sanitize water and catalyze bromine. It is often used to shock water without the use of chlorine.

Precipitate. A compound that is or becomes insoluble and falls out of solution; also, to fall out of solution.

Pressure differential. The difference in pressure between two or more actions of a hydraulic system, such as the difference in pressure between the inlet flow and outlet flow of a pump or filter.

Pressure gauge. A device that registers the pressure in a water or air system. Pressure is usually measured in pounds per square inch (psi).

Prime. The process of preparing a pump for operation by displacing the air on the suction side of the circulation system with water.

Pump. A motor-driven device that moves water.

Reagent. A liquid or dry chemical formulated to create a reaction (usually a color change) when it comes into contact with a particular compound in water. Used for water testing.

Recirculating system. The complete water filtration system, consisting of pipes, pump, strainer, filter, and skimmer.

Return line. The line through which water is discharged into the pool or spa; also called an *inlet*.

Sanitizer. Any chemical compound added to water that kills bacteria. Some sanitizers also oxidize organic material.

Scale. Deposits of calcium carbonate.

Sequestering agent. A chemical that causes small particles of metals to combine so that they are large enough to be trapped by a pool or spa filter.

Shock treatment. The addition of pool or spa sanitizers in a larger-than-normal amount in order to eliminate unusual water conditions, such as infestations of algae, the presence of chloramines, or colored water. *See also* Superchlorination.

Shotcrete. A premix of sand, concrete, and water used to create a pool or spa shell. It is applied through an air-powered nozzle.

Sight glass. A clear glass or plastic section of pipe that permits viewing of the water in the line. It allows one to see when the water is clear, for example, during the backwashing of a filter.

Skimmer. A device that removes leaves and other floating debris from the water surface by drawing water through it.

Slurry. A watery mixture. Usually refers to the mixture of diatomaceous earth and water that's used to coat the grids in a DE filter.

Soda ash. *See* Sodium carbonate.

Sodium bicarbonate. In swimming pools, sodium bicarbonate (also known as *baking soda*) is commonly used to raise the alkalinity of the water. Unlike sodium carbonate, sodium bicarbonate does not raise the pH noticeably.

Sodium bisulfate. A compound of sodium and acid sulfate that can be used to bring down the pH in water through an increase of hydrogen ions. Also known as *dry acid*.

Sodium carbonate. A dry chemical (also known as *soda ash*) used to increase the pH of pool water

Soft water. Water is considered soft if it has less than 50 ppm (parts per million) of calcium carbonate and less than 30 ppm of calcium chloride. The pH can be rather unstable in soft-water areas, but an alkaline chlorine donor such as calcium hypochlorite will help increase hardness, as will the addition of calcium chloride.

Stabilizer. A water conditioner, such as cyanuric acid, added to pool water to extend the effective life of chlorine by protecting it from the dissipating effects of sunlight.

Strainer pot. In a pump, a filter that prevents large debris, such as leaves, from being pulled into the pool's circulation system.

Superchlorination. The addition of larger-than-normal amounts of chlorine, especially during periods of excessive heat, rainfall, or pool use, to convert chloramines into free available chlorine by destroying ammonia.

Telepole. A metal or fiberglass pole used with pool and spa cleaning tools that extends to twice its original length.

Therm. A unit of measurement for natural gas. It equals 100,000 Btus/hour of heat.

Total alkalinity (TA). The measurement of all alkaline chemicals in pool water. When TA is too high, the pH resists adjustment to the desired range. When TA is too low, it is difficult to maintain the pH within the desired range.

Total dissolved solids (TDS). The amount of conductive chemicals in pool water. You cannot see these "solids" because they are dissolved, but this does not stop them from corroding metal parts (such as pumps, pipes, and filters). They are made up mostly of chlorides and sulfates. Chlorides can accumulate with long-term use of sodium hypochlorite. Regular addition of alum-based clarifiers (aluminum sulfate) and dry acid (sodium bisulfate) can increase sulfate levels. Periodic backwashing and water replacement are the best ways to control TDS.

Total dynamic head. The total amount of resistance (measured in feet) created by pipes, fittings, and equipment in the circulation system.

Trichlor. Short for *trichlor*oisocyanuric acid. A stabilized chlorine donor usually sold in the form of slowly dissolving tablets of 91 percent available chlorine. When dissolved in water, trichlor dissociates (splits up) into hypochlorous acid (free chlorine) and cyanuric acid.

Turnover rate. The time it takes for a pool or spa's circulation system to pass through the filter a volume of water equal to the amount of water contained in the pool or spa. Usually expressed in hours.

Vacuum wall fitting. A fitting in the pool wall below the waterline for attaching the hose of a pool vacuum (suction) hose. In some pools, the vacuum fitting is located in the skimmer box.

Venturi. A short tube with a constricted passage that increases the velocity and lowers the pressure of a gas or fluid sent through it. It can be adjusted to regulate mixtures.

Weir. The hinged plate in the "throat" or inlet of a skimmer box.

Index

Page numbers in *italic* indicate illustrations; those in **bold** indicate tables.

OTHER STOREY TITLES
YOU WILL ENJOY

Deckscaping by Barbara W. Ellis. Use your deck more in every season. The author suggests surfaces, lighting, plantings, and furniture — from simple to elaborate — and gives tips on maintenance. 176 pages. ISBN 1-58017-408-6 (paper with French flaps); ISBN 1-58017-459-0 (hardcover).

The Flower Gardener's Bible by Lewis and Nancy Hill. Friendly, indispensable, and written with wit and authority, this book is painstakingly thorough and stunningly photographed. Covers every facet of growing perennials, annuals, bulbs, wildflowers, small trees, vines and shrubs for season-long color and beauty. 384 pages. ISBN 1-58017-462-0 (paperback); ISBN 1-58017-463-9 (hardcover).

Grasses by Nancy J. Ondra. A complete introduction to using ornamental grasses in combination with perennials, annuals, shrubs, and other garden plants. Beautiful full-color photographs. 144 pages. Paper with French flaps. ISBN 1-58017-423-X.

Poolscaping by Catriona Tudor Erler. Inspiring ideas and practical advice on how to make your swimming pool a lovely, welcoming centerpiece of your property. Illustrated with beautiful full-color photographs of outstanding poolscapes. 208 pages. Paper with French flaps. ISBN 1-58017-385-3.

Outdoor Water Features by Alan and Gill Bridgewater. Add the sparkle and serenity of water to your landscape with these 16 functional and beautiful projects. 128 pages. Paperback. ISBN 1-58017-334-9.

Shady Retreats by Barbara Ellis. Most flowers and vegetables love the sun, but gardeners who tend them crave the shade. This beautifully illustrated book provides detailed plans for 20 gardens with shade as a theme, easy-to-read blueprints, plants lists, and suggestions on how to bring color into the shade. 192 pages. Paperback. ISBN 1-58017-472-8.

Stonescaping by Jan Kowalczewski Whitner. Practical and detailed directions for incorporating the beauty and strength of stone into more than 20 Asian, European, and contemporary home garden designs. 168 pages. Paperback. ISBN 0-88266-755-6.

Waterscaping by Judy Glattstein. Whether you are installing a commercially produced pond, own property with an existing stream or pond, or face the challenges of landscaping a "too wet" area of your yard, this book covers everything you need to know about water gardening. 192 pages. Paperback. ISBN 0-88266-606-1.

These and other books from Storey Publishing are available wherever quality books are sold or by calling 1-800-441-5700. Visit us at www.storey.com.